the gluten-free TABLE

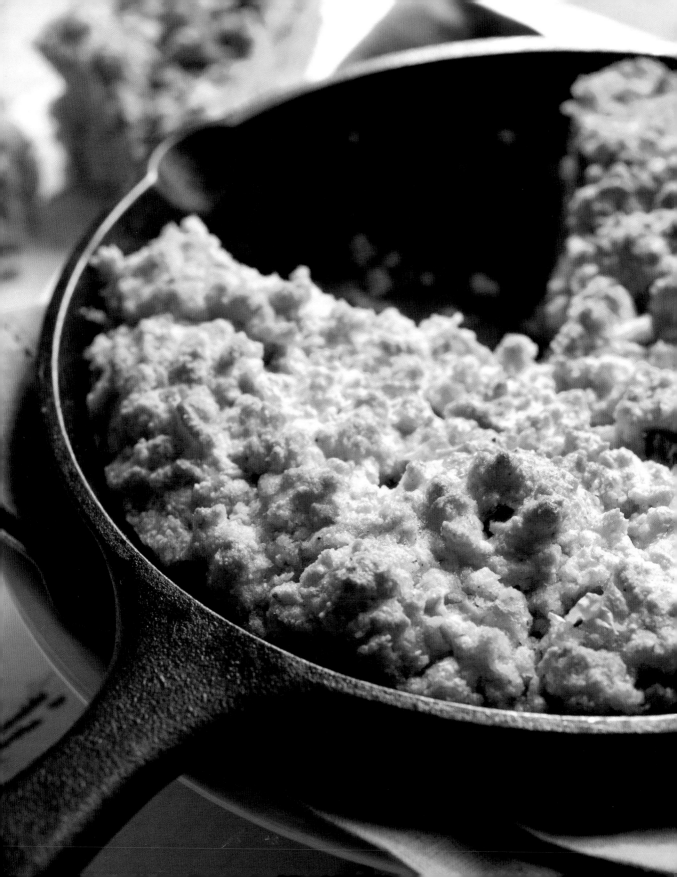

the gluten-free
TABLE

· *The Lagasse Girls* ·

SHARE THEIR FAVORITE MEALS

Jilly Lagasse & Jessie Lagasse Swanson

FOREWORD BY EMERIL LAGASSE

GRAND CENTRAL
Life & Style
NEW YORK · BOSTON

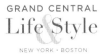

Copyright © 2012 by Jessie Lagasse Swanson and Jilly Lagasse

All rights reserved. In accordance with the U.S. Copyright Act of 1976, the scanning, uploading, and electronic sharing of any part of this book without the permission of the publisher constitutes unlawful piracy and theft of the author's intellectual property. If you would like to use material from the book (other than for review purposes), prior written permission must be obtained by contacting the publisher at permissions@hbgusa.com. Thank you for your support of the author's rights.

Grand Central Life & Style
Hachette Book Group
237 Park Avenue
New York, NY 10017
www.HachetteBookGroup.com

Printed in the United States of America

Wor

Originally published in hardcover by Grand Central Life & Style.

First trade edition: April 2014

10 9 8 7 6 5 4 3 2 1

Grand Central Life & Style is an imprint of Grand Central Publishing.

The Grand Central Life & Style name and logo are trademarks of Hachette Book Group, Inc.

The Hachette Speakers Bureau provides a wide range of authors for speaking events. To find out more, go to www.hachettespeakersbureau.com or call (866) 376-6591.

The publisher is not responsible for websites (or their content) that are not owned by the publisher.

The Library of Congress has cataloged the hardcover edition as follows:
Lagasse, Jilly.
    The gluten-free table : the Lagasse girls share their favorite meals / by Jilly Lagasse and Jessie Lagasse Swanson.
      p. cm.
    ISBN 978-1-4555-1688-9 (hardback)
  1. Gluten-free diet—Recipes.   I. Lagasse Swanson, Jessie.
II. Title.
    RM237.86.L34 2012
    641.3—dc23

                                              2012013270

ISBN 978-1-4555-1687-2 (pbk.)

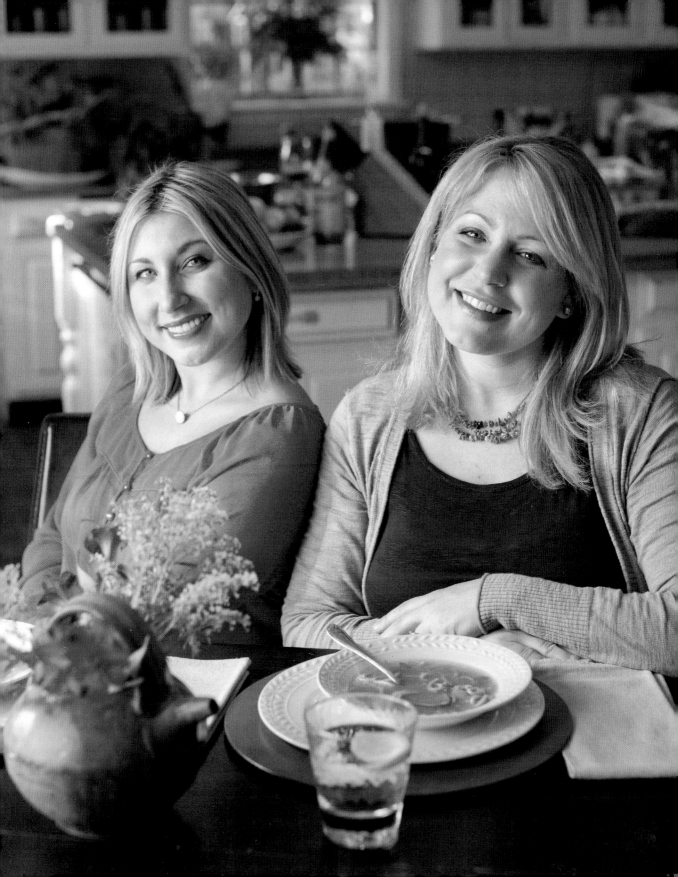

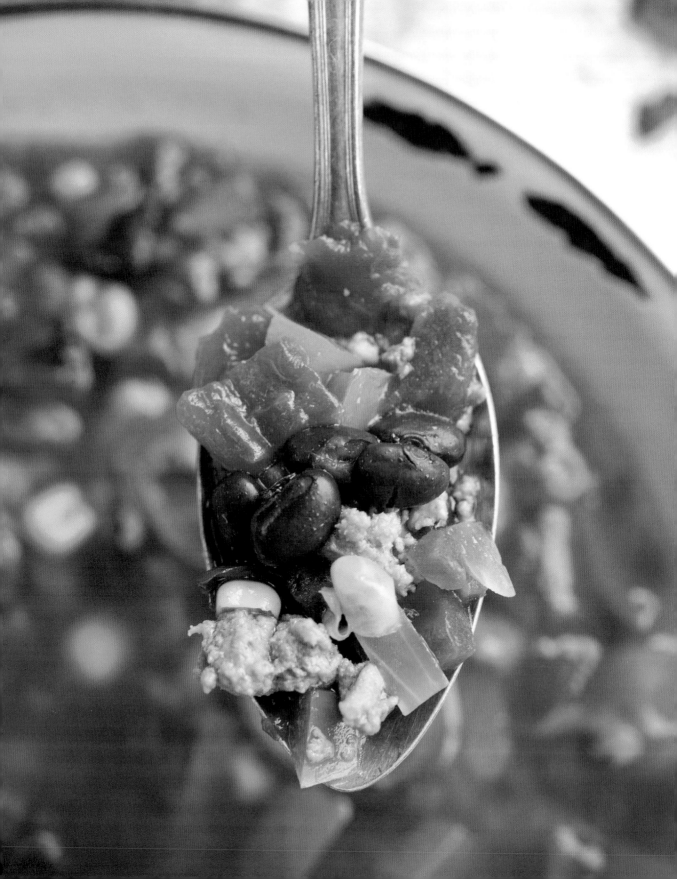

contents

foreword

Sharing a family meal, whether it be a casual dinner at home or dinner out to celebrate a special occasion, is something I consider one of the most sacred and important experiences a family shares.

"Cook together, eat together, and be together" is something I learned from my mother, Hilda, and not only did it influence me to make cooking my profession, but it also meant that the kitchen would be the center of my home when I had a family of my own.

Preparing and enjoying food together was a priority in my house, so when two of my daughters had to follow restrictive diets, it was quite a change. First and foremost, my biggest concern was their health, and the furthest thing from my mind was that what they were eating could be causing them pain and making their symptoms worse! I had never heard of celiac disease, so you can imagine my surprise when I learned that the only successful treatment was to totally eliminate wheat from their diet. It was hard for me to wrap my head around no more pasta for Jilly (my spaghetti Bolognese partner) and no more of Jessie's favorite pizzas. Once the girls began following a gluten-free diet, the mystery ailments that had been troubling them for years disappeared. It quickly became

obvious to me that this was something very real and very serious, and that as a chef and a dad, I needed to get with the program!

Fast-forward to today. We now know that 1 in 133 people have celiac disease. Gluten intolerance is one of the most common, yet misunderstood and underdiagnosed diseases. Although much has been discovered since Jilly's initial diagnosis many years ago, one simple truth we can't get away from is that a gluten-free diet is the only medically accepted treatment for this disease. I've seen food trends come and go during my years as a chef, but I'm here to tell you that this is no trend, folks; this is a serious reality for people living with gluten intolerance and celiac disease. And, hey, even folks who just want to be healthier and feel better can benefit from a gluten-free regimen.

At first a gluten-free diet might seem restrictive and hard to follow. I remember being so puzzled as to what I could create that was wheat-free but still delicious. Although it was challenging at first, once we all put our heads

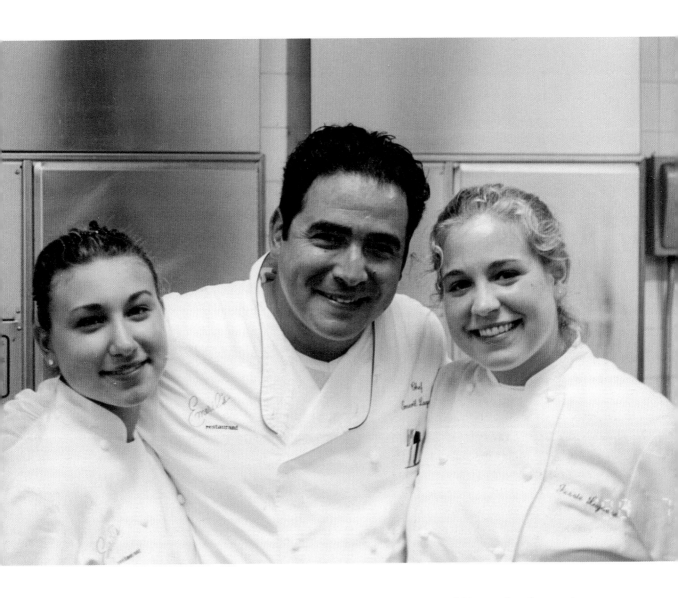

together and focused on what *is* "allowed," all sorts of options opened up for us. The girls have followed me around the kitchen from an early age, and they are naturals in that environment. They have inspired me with their creative, gluten-free takes on our family favorites. I am proud to see what my daughters have created together here, and I know that they are just as excited to share these recipes with you! I think they are simple yet delicious reinterpretations of family favorites that will provide you with gluten-free choices you've never imagined. So dig in and enjoy these amazing recipes around a gluten-free family table.

Emeril J. Lagasse III

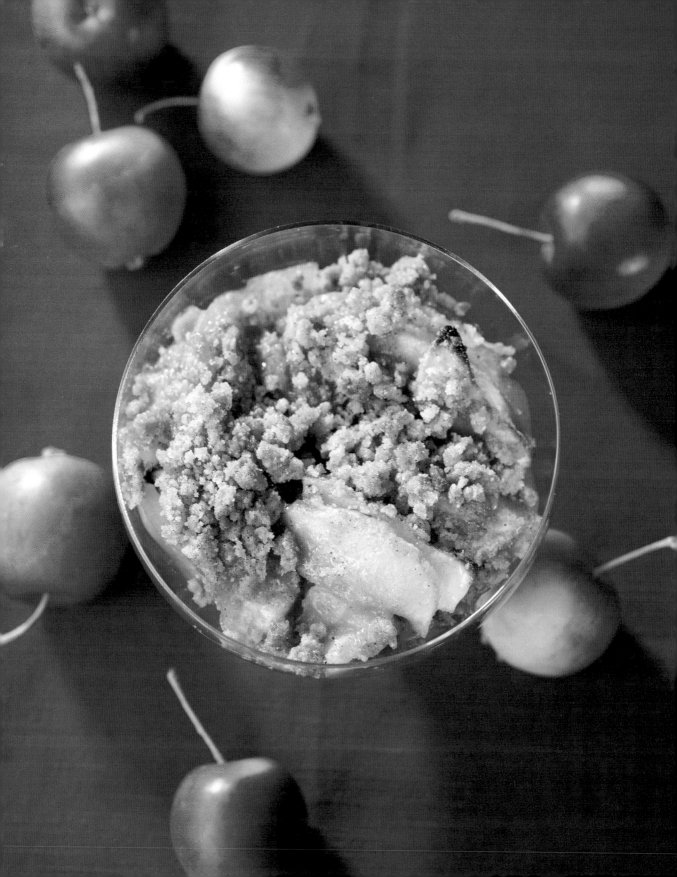

the gluten-free TABLE

introduction

Growing up with our father, Emeril Lagasse, we were instilled with a love of cooking and an appreciation for food from as early as we can remember. Creating pleasant food memories, and sharing laughter around the dinner table, has always been a focus in our lives.

It was our dad who taught both of us to cook, simple dishes at first—like the scrambled eggs he taught Jessie to make when she was five years old, or the simple butter cookie recipe he shared with Jilly's elementary school class—and then on to more complex flavors and dishes. It was so easy, and so natural—a father sharing his acquired knowledge and passion for food, and passing down long-cherished family recipes to his daughters.

Until one day we literally couldn't eat them anymore. In 2001, after traditional physicians had failed to alleviate her persistent symptoms, Jessie visited a naturopathic doctor and was diagnosed with a gluten sensitivity. Sure enough, after she'd identified the culprit and modified her diet, her symptoms disappeared. Jilly was diagnosed with celiac disease in February of 2004. She had struggled health-wise for years and was constantly misdiagnosed with everything from irritable bowel syndrome to iron deficiency. It wasn't until she visited a new doctor in London that the answer was revealed. After hearing her symptoms, he suggested a simple blood test that confirmed celiac disease. Once she'd switched to a strictly gluten-free diet, Jilly's life improved by leaps and bounds. Her illnesses started to fade, her health quickly returned, and she felt something she hadn't in a long time: energy!

We'll be honest: it wasn't always easy adjusting to a gluten-free lifestyle. We needed to change the way we ate and the way we cooked and to learn to plan ahead and pay attention to ingredients in ways we never had before. However, our quality of life improved so dramatically that we saw our diagnoses as a blessing, not a curse. The generally accepted statistic is that 1 in every 133 people have celiac disease. Yet, as many as 97 percent don't even know it! This number does not include the thousands of others who are gluten intolerant but do not have full-fledged celiac disease.

Happy to be on the road to health, we started thinking about food in a new way, focusing on fresh vegetables and whole grains,

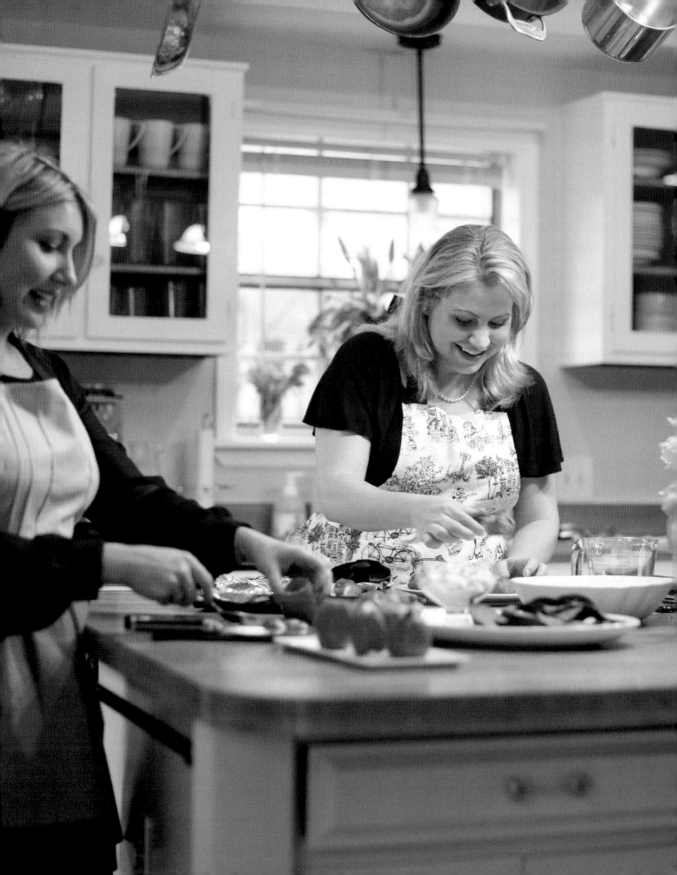

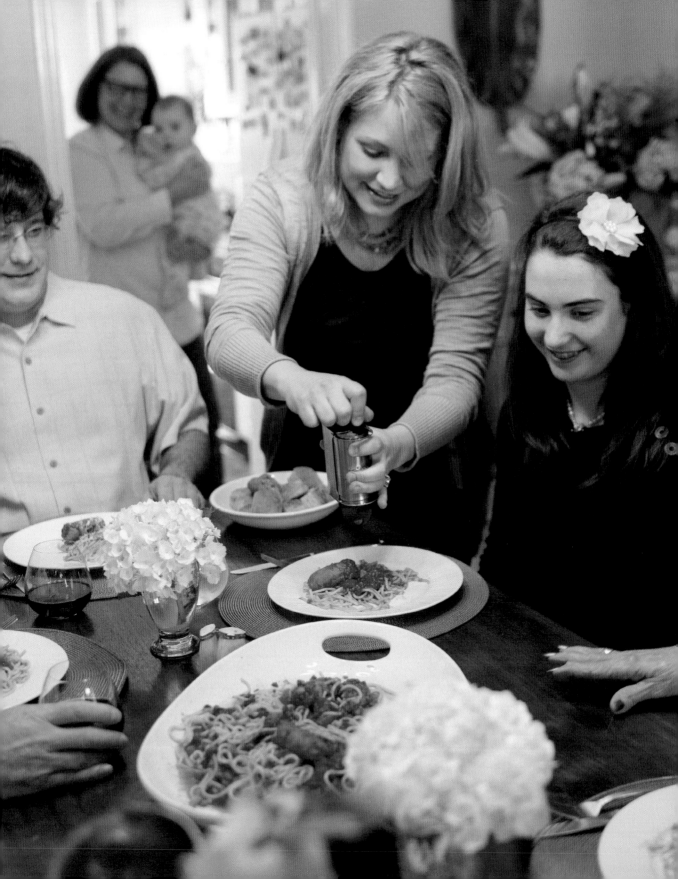

meals we could make using flour substitutes that replaced gluten as a binding ingredient. It was challenging, and at first our father was hesitant to take our new diet seriously. After all, in 2001 when Jessie was first diagnosed, the term "gluten-free" was not very common. As time progressed, however, our father became more educated about the subject and now routinely offers gluten-free foods at our family Sunday dinners. He even makes gluten-free gumbo, which is one of our favorite dishes!

A traditional New Orleans gumbo, of course, relies on a roux—a flour and fat base used to thicken many soups and sauces (and a common base in this book). Requiring flour as a key component, roux were an early challenge to learning to cook and eat gluten-free and also an unavoidable one, as many of our favorite recipes relied on them. It took us years to find adequate wheat substitutes that not only provided the same consistency as a traditional roux but also tasted similar. Now there are a myriad of gluten-free flour mixes that meet these standards, and an explosion of higher-quality and delicious gluten-free foods in the marketplace. We couldn't be more excited!

This sense of excitement and newfound possibility led us to the idea of writing a cookbook. We'd both experienced the frustration and sadness, early on, of wanting familiar foods but not being able to find an adequate gluten-free recipe, or recipe component, to re-create them. Imagine never again being able to indulge in buttercream-frosted birthday cake or brick-oven pizza—the stakes were high, to say the least. Finding the right gluten-free product was so paramount, the right gluten-free recipe so thrilling, that e-mails, tips, and suggestions began flying constantly back and forth. Coming up with

full-flavored, nearly indistinguishable versions of the hearty foods we grew up with, and some of the more aromatic, complex dishes we'd come to crave as adults, became a personal challenge, then an obsession, and finally, once we'd tackled many of our gluten-free bugaboos (including that dastardly roux), a true joy. As soon as we got more comfortable with cooking gluten-free, we embarked on a five-year journey to redevelop and perfect our

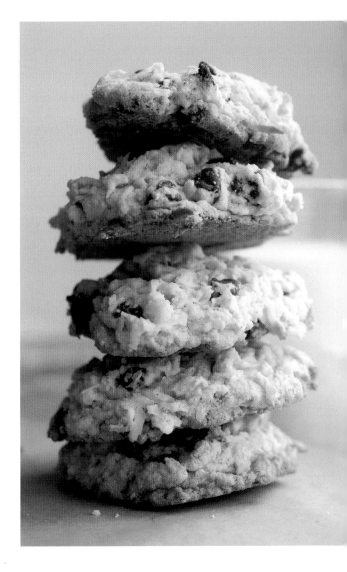

own favorite recipes into tasty, celiac-friendly alternatives, our only hope for making other people as delighted as we were each time one of our recipes worked. That characteristic, too, we owe to our father. He gets more joy out of seeing people enjoying good food than any other person we know. It's contagious, in a way, and another reason why we decided to write this book—to share our joy of this food with others and hopefully bring you, our readers, the same pleasure!

Although there are a lot more gluten-free products on the market now than there used to be, there are still many times when a good home-cooked gluten-free meal or snack is preferred. This cookbook is intended to provide a well-balanced base of recipes that can add flavor and enjoyment to the menus of even the pickiest or most demanding of gluten-free eaters. That's not to say we require or would even have time to make everything from scratch! If there is a gluten-free cracker or pizza crust you really like, by all means substitute it in place of our homemade or referenced version. The same goes for any of the recommended brands we include in our recipes. You'll notice we often include our father's spices in our recipes. It's not that we are shamelessly plugging our dad's products; it's simply that we learned how to cook using them, and now they are our go-to spices. You can use any Cajun spice you want and still get a tasty result. Cooking, as we well know, is personal, and we hope that these recipes inspire you to add your own unique touches as you see fit.

This book has been such a wonderful journey for us both, and one that has spanned years and found us covered in every kind of gluten-free flour imaginable. Anyone who knows us would agree that we are two very different people with very diverse preferences, but creating the book together has given us an opportunity to explore that uniqueness while working together for a common goal. There are traditional, time-tested family recipes here as well as slightly more gourmet fare, for when you're entertaining or want to try something new. Recipes run the gamut from classic New Orleans favorites to more conservative New England staples to unique ethnic specialties with many different flavors, textures, and ingredients. Through it all, though, runs the consistent theme of delicious, easy-to-prepare gluten-free recipes that will appeal to even the most disparate palates. There really is something for everyone here.

The most significant lesson we have learned years into a gluten-free diet is that such restrictions require flexibility and creativity. This is nothing to be scared of but rather a part of gluten-free eating that should be embraced and explored. There are many ways to enjoy foods that taste just as good as, if not better than, their gluten-filled counterparts. The recipes in this book provide a starting point. With a little inventiveness and perseverance, you can find joy and triumph in a gluten-free diet and won't feel like you're missing a thing. Best of luck to you!

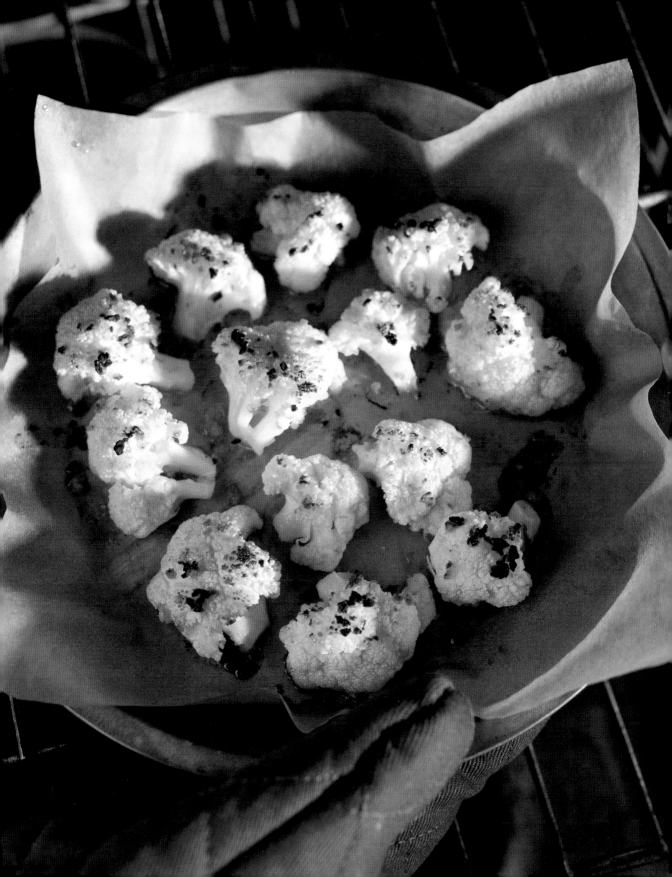

living gluten-free and lovin' it

Over the last few years, gluten-free eating has caused quite a fuss in homes, retail outlets, and restaurants across the country. All we can say is, *"It's about time!"*

We have struggled with and triumphed over gluten-free diets for years, and we are so thrilled the general population is finally taking notice! Before we get into the meat and potatoes of our recipes, we thought it'd be helpful to lay some groundwork in this chapter. We'll talk about the ins and outs of a gluten-free kitchen and lifestyle, including foods you can have and what you'll need to avoid, how to have a safe, working kitchen for both the gluten-free and non-gluten-free members of your household, and how to stock your very own gluten-free pantry. You will also find a brief list of resources at the end of the book that can connect you to groups doing great things for the gluten-free set as well as links to retailers stocking some of our favorite gluten-free ingredients. Interested? Please read on!

Living a gluten-free life is of utter importance when you have celiac disease or a gluten sensitivity, but that doesn't have to mean you live a life eating bland, boring, or tasteless food. We hope to show you what a delicious little culinary adventure you are about to embark upon. The pleasure of cooking and the enjoyment of tasting new foods in a new way is such a wonderful part of living life. And with this book, you will see that being diagnosed with this disease or intolerance doesn't have to change that.

Let's start by talking briefly about some statistics and theories. Recent studies show that at least 3 million Americans, or 1 in every 133 people, have celiac disease. Yet only 1 in 4,700 is properly diagnosed! As you probably know, getting a diagnosis can be quite challenging.

Generally, we think it is underdiagnosed for a few different reasons. Some studies suggest celiac disease mostly affects people of European descent, in particular northern European people. Because of the amalgamation of ethnicities in our melting pot of a country, there is no one group that stands out as having a significant undiagnosed problem. Physicians aren't finding any correlation between a certain ethnic group and symptoms, and no warning bells are going off. More significantly, generally speaking it seems like many doctors in the US just aren't as clear or knowledgeable about celiac disease and gluten sensitivity as they are in some other countries. Physicians, therefore, often attribute the disease's common symptoms to another illness or a slew of illnesses instead.

Fortunately, as we are seeing now, awareness of the disease is increasing every day, due largely to the seeming increase in the number of people affected with celiac-type symptoms. Celiac disease, also known as *celiac sprue*, is a hereditary (genetically predisposed) autoimmune disease of the small intestine that makes it impossible for people to digest gluten, the protein found in wheat, barley, rye, spelt, triticale, and kamut.

It affects how the vitamins and nutrients from the food you eat are absorbed by your body. Your small intestine is lined with villi, tiny little fingerlike sponges that absorb all the nutrients you put into your body and help transfer these nutrients into the bloodstream. When you have celiac disease and eat foods containing gluten, the gluten protein injures the villi and makes them unable to absorb the much-needed vitamins and nutrients in food.

It's important to remember that people can have celiac disease and not show any symptoms. Common symptoms include stomach issues such as recurring abdominal bloating, cramping, and chronic diarrhea. Other symptoms, including fatigue, headaches, and joint pain, can also occur.

And one person's symptoms may be very different from another's.

Once you get your diagnosis, it's time to begin treatment. After following a strict gluten-

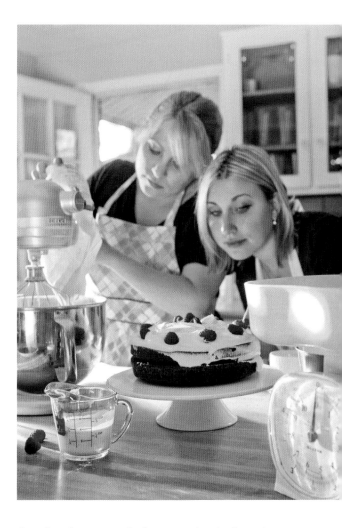

free diet for a period of time, individuals with gluten sensitivity might, under the guidance of their doctors, eventually be able to reintroduce small amounts of gluten-containing foods into their diet. However, at present the only treatment for celiac disease is adhering to a strict gluten-free diet for the remainder of your life. Initially, that sounds tragic and depressing, but it doesn't have to be. With this book, we will show you that a gluten-free life doesn't have to bring tears to your eyes and sadness to you at the grocery store. Quite the opposite, it can be a wonderful, delicious journey!

gluten-free shopping

So go ahead and ask us: "Hey, ladies, what can I eat now?" We are here to tell you, *loads*! You're going to start to realize that when you grocery shop now, you'll most often be in the outer perimeter of the store—fresh produce, meats, seafood, and dairy. You'll, of course, venture into the inner aisles for other staples like rice, beans, sauces, even some frozen foods. But you can say good-bye to most of the processed, refined products that may have been a part of your pre-gluten-free diet.

Even though there are tons of options, you will *have* to become a master of reading and checking every label on every item you buy! Almost like a Columbo of food labels, you will have to learn to dissect and translate ingredients and contents to ferret out any sneaky sources of gluten. Luckily, many companies are beginning to print "gluten-free" on their packaging, and this surely makes the process easier. But you still have to be vigilant and thorough because gluten can hide itself in so many things and disguise itself under many different names.

Gluten can be hiding in preservatives, food stabilizers, malt flavoring, modified food starch, hydrolyzed vegetable or plant protein (HVP/HPP, made from wheat protein), and thickeners used to "enhance" food. It can even be found in some medications, vitamins, Communion wafers, and even the glue on envelopes.

Here is a list of items for which you'll have to read the labels, as they can contain wheat and gluten:

Creamy soups or sauces (Why are they thick? A wheat-flour roux or thickener with gluten?)

Bouillon or stock cubes

Premade marinades and salad dressings

Cheese sauces, pasta sauces

Communion wafers

Some potato and corn tortilla chips (if seasoned)

Licorice

Some deli meat/cold cuts, hot dogs, self-basting turkey

Some salamis and sausages (Wheat can be used to bind and thicken them up.)

Store-bought meatballs (often contain bread crumbs)

Gravy and gravy mixes (usually thickened with wheat flour)

Some barbecue sauces

Store-bought dips and dip mixes

Some French fries (Though potatoes are safe, some can be breaded or seasoned with a wheat-flour blend.)

Imitation crabmeat

Matzo crackers, as well as most crackers

Packaged dry soup mixes

Packaged rice mixes

Some spice blends

Soy sauce (made from wheat flour)

Beer, ale, all malt beverages

Malt vinegar

When one considers just how many foods are out there for our consumption, this list is not overly oppressive, right? We are obliged to say, though, that the preceding list and any of the ones that follow are *not* all-inclusive. Please use them as a starting point from which to create your own personal "do" and "don't" food lists, but don't feel as though you must confine your gluten-free diet to those items mentioned. To do so would be to vastly restrict your options, and you'll be missing out on a lot of other gluten-free possibilities we just might not have had the space to discuss.

eating gluten-free

Now that we've talked about some of the gluten-free diet "don'ts," let's briefly look at some of the wonderful things you can still feed your body—and there are many!

• You can have any breads, cakes, cookies, pastas, noodles, cereals, and crackers made from the following: corn, rice, soy, arrowroot, potato starch, tapioca starch, gram or chickpea flour, bean flour, rice bran, cornmeal, polenta, buckwheat, millet, flax, sorghum, amaranth, and quinoa.

• You can have all fresh, frozen, or canned varieties of vegetables. Just make sure to buy them plain, unseasoned, and without a premade sauce.

• All fruits and fruit juices are safe, but check the labels of premade fruit pie fillings, some fruit cups, and dried fruit just to be safe.

• Most dairy products are usually fair game, too, so all milk and milk products, cheeses, and yogurts are generally safe. Check labels on certain flavored yogurts, ice creams, frozen yogurts, creamers, malted milk and flavored milk drinks and smoothies, and margarine.

• Meat, poultry, fish, shellfish, and eggs are safe. Check labels of prepackaged deli meats, premarinated items, hot dogs, sausages, meatballs, and canned meats.

• All beans, nuts, dried peas, lentils, soybeans, peanut butter, and almond butter are safe.

• Generally, all sugar, honey, jams and jellies, hard candy, plain chocolate, coconut, marshmallows, meringues, molasses, and most spices are gluten-free, too.

• Interestingly, lots of ethnic foods are almost always naturally gluten-free. Many Indian, Thai, and Vietnamese foods utilize rice, bean flours, coconut milk, fresh produce, meats or seafood, and wonderful spices. Introducing this variety into your regular humdrum diet adds a tasty new dimension that we really recommend you explore a bit.

Let's move on to beverages next.

• Most tea, coffee, and carbonated drinks are usually gluten-free, as are some protein drinks made with whey protein.

• Alcoholic beverages can be tricky, so let's discuss these in a bit more detail. Beers of most kinds are usually a no-no, as they are made with wheat. In the past few years, though, several companies have begun distributing gluten-free beers. While slightly different in taste, most versions are very good approximations of the gluten-laden original and deserve a try.

• Generally speaking, almost all wines and distilled alcohols like gin and vodka are safe. To avoid confusion, though, here is a comprehensive list of those alcohols that are gluten-free:

Armagnac (made from grapes, so this is okay)

Bourbon (Maker's Mark only)

Champagne (contains yeast, though, so avoid if you have yeast sensitivity)

Cider (usually made from apples, but check for barley)

Cognac (made from grapes, so this is okay)

Gin (all except Bombay Sapphire and Beefeater, which contain licorice)

Grappa

Kahlúa

Kirschwasser (a cherry brandy)

Margarita mix (Jose Cuervo, Mr & Mrs T)

Margaritas (Skinnygirl)

Martinis (Club Vodka Martini and Extra Dry Martini are from corn and grapes, so okay)

Mead (from honey)

Ouzo (grape and anise are safe)

Rum, light and dark

Sake (fermented rice and koji)

Scotch whiskey

Sparkling wine (see also Champagne, above)

Tequila

Vermouth (from grapes)

Vodka (Stoli)

Wine coolers

Wines, including cooking wines, sherry, and port

See, it is possible to follow a gluten-free lifestyle *and* still have a beer or cocktail!

the gluten-free pantry

Now that we know some of the major foods you can and cannot have while adhering to a gluten-free diet, let's look at what we recommend every gluten-free pantry should contain. We'll give it to you in list form, so it's easier to decipher.

For Baking

Gluten-free flour blends or gluten-free all-purpose baking mix

Almond meal/flour

Amaranth flour

Buckwheat flour

Chickpea flour (aka gram flour)

Corn flour, cornmeal, cornstarch

Millet flour

Rice flour

Sorghum flour

Baking powder and baking soda (gluten-free)

Xanthan gum

Guar gum

Honey, molasses, agave syrup

Applesauce (all natural unsweetened)

Fruit preserves (good quality)

Shredded coconut

Coconut milk

Condensed milk

Sugar (light and dark brown, granulated, baker's [superfine], confectioner's)

Chocolate (good-quality milk, dark, white)

Dried fruit (cherries, cranberries, etc.)

Nuts (walnuts, pecans, peanuts)

Salt

Ghee (clarified butter)

Vanilla extract (all natural)

Spices (all-natural cloves, cinnamon sticks, vanilla bean pods, cardamom, nutmeg)

Pastas, Cereals, Grains, and Dried Legumes

Gluten-free pastas (any blend of corn, rice, quinoa and any brand, shape you prefer, including lasagna noodles)

Gluten-free rice noodles (vermicelli and pad Thai–cut rice noodles, bean thread noodles)

Gluten-free oats and oatmeal

Gluten-free cereals

Corn tortillas

Corn grits and polenta

Quinoa

Rices (brown, white, jasmine, basmati, wild)

Rice cakes (Plain, unsalted are best.)

Dried beans (red kidney, black, black-eyed peas, adzukis)

Dried peas and lentils

Canned and Bottled Goods, Sauces, and Seasonings

Canned chopped tomatoes, tomato paste, tomato sauce

Canned corn, olives, hearts of palm

Canned beans (red kidney, black, black-eyed peas, adzukis)

Vinegars (apple cider, red, white, balsamic, cooking sherry)

Oils (olive, coconut, vegetable, sunflower, avocado)

Peanut butter, almond butter (all natural)

Fruit preserves (all natural)

Salsas

Hot sauces (Tapatío, Tabasco, Sriracha, Vietnamese chili and garlic sauce)

Thai fish sauce

Thai-style sweet chili dipping sauce

Tamari (gluten-free soy sauce)

Condiments (mayonnaise, mustards)

Spices and seasonings (all natural)

Gluten-free stock or stock cubes

Curry pastes (Thai green or red, Indian mild, or Madras curry paste)

With a pantry stocked like this, the possibilities of great-tasting, nutritious, and delicious gluten-free meals are endless. So get cooking!

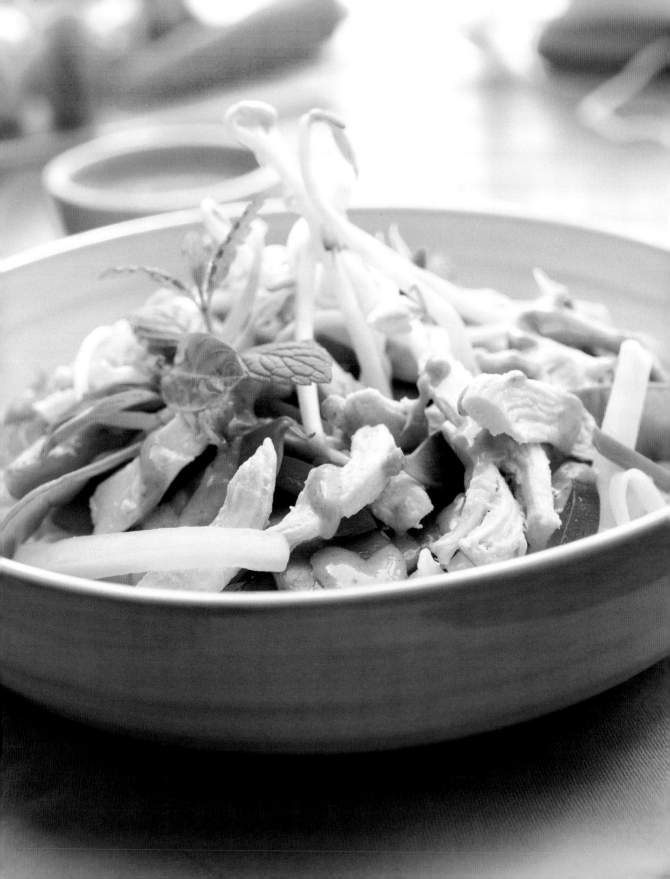

cooking gluten-free

Oh, but wait—you're wondering how to keep the foods needed for your gluten-free family member separate from those of the rest of the gluten-filled household? Let's talk cross-contamination, then, shall we? Cross-contamination occurs when gluten comes in contact with gluten-free foods or products and, in turn, "contaminates" them. This can happen in several ways, unfortunately. Every shared surface, be it a toaster or even a butter knife, runs the risk of cross-contamination. Here is a list of some you may or may not be aware of:

Shared Oil in Deep Fryers or Frying Pans

Hooray! Gluten-free individuals are still able to eat (most) French fries as well as some brands of gluten-free chicken nuggets and breaded fish products. However, if the fryer and/or oil in which the gluten-free versions are cooked is also the same fryer and/or oil being used to cook traditional glutenous foods, cross-contamination is possible. Ideally, there should be separate fryers for gluten and gluten-free foods.

BBQ Grills

Another sneaky one to watch out for, the home barbecue grill can contaminate even the best gluten-free food. If meats marinated in a gluten-laden sauce have been grilled on the same surface as a gluten-free meat, cross-contamination can occur. Make sure the grill is properly cleaned of all other products before cooking any gluten-free items.

Toasters and Toaster Ovens

Again, if toasters are shared with non-gluten-free products, cross-contamination is possible. It may not be ideal to have two separate toasters or toaster ovens, so we recommend getting a four-slice toaster and divvying up sides to the gluten-frees and the regulars. This will minimize contamination without requiring a second kitchen just for your kids' toast!

Cutting Boards

It's very important to wash cutting boards *very* well in hot, soapy water if they are shared by gluten and gluten-free foods. As silly as it seems, we highly recommend having two separate cutting boards in the kitchen, one dedicated to gluten-free and one to non-gluten-free food preparation.

Utensils, Cutlery, Pots, and Pans

All have to be washed thoroughly if shared to avoid cross-contamination. Also, do *not* share a pot of boiling water to cook both gluten-free and traditional pasta. If sharing the pot can't be avoided, cook the gluten-free version first to avoid contaminating it as much as possible.

Shared Condiments

Shared butter or margarine, spreads, cream cheese, jars of jams or jellies, jars of peanut butters, almond butters, mayonnaise, and mustards can *all* easily become cross-contaminated if shared when preparing food. If you want to have only one jar of each of these items, we recommend instituting a "clean spoon" rule. Always use a clean spoon to scoop out your condiment. Put it into a separate small bowl and use that bowl from which to spread it. This way, the gluten-covered butter knife never goes into the mayonnaise or jelly jar.

Baking Equipment

Flour sifters, measuring scales, measuring cups, electric beaters, mixers, baking trays, and any other baking accoutrement should be thoroughly cleaned in hot, soapy water if they are shared with gluten-laden baking processes.

Colanders

When draining pasta, using the same colander for gluten and gluten-free pastas creates a high risk of cross-contamination because real wheat pasta can get stuck in the holes of the colander and contaminate your lovely gluten-free version. Again, if you can, invest in two separate colanders for your home. As tricky as it is to get a colander really, really clean (you know what we mean), we think having two is worth it!

Dried Peas, Lentils, and Beans

Especially if bought from bulk bins, some pesky gluten-laden grains can easily get mixed up with the other products. We prefer to buy separate bags of these ingredients just to be safe. Either way, always make sure to sift and sort through your purchased product and pick out anything that looks suspicious. This is not a 100 percent fail-safe method, but it's better than nothing!

Don't be too hard on yourself, okay? It is virtually impossible to have a perfectly safe home kitchen environment if you are preparing both gluten-full and gluten-free foods. You are realistically going to have to do the best you can. However, this list of tips can make a big difference, and we strongly advocate your implementing some or all of them if you can. Your villi will thank you!

eating out

Lots of these tips are also fair game for restaurants. People suffering from gluten sensitivities or celiac disease want to eat out sometimes, too. But with all the dos and don'ts and the fear of cross-contamination, finding a safe, gluten-free meal out can be daunting. According to celiac-disease.com, people with celiac disease dine out 80 percent less than they used to before diagnosis, and it's no wonder. It can be so confusing and overwhelming to find a safe, tasty meal at a restaurant. But it is getting easier and easier every day, thanks to the growing awareness of gluten issues and to the skyrocketing market demand for gluten-free fare (yay capitalism!).

Some restaurants now even offer specific gluten-free meals on their menus. Others will be happy to construct a safe version of your desired entrée if you ask. But *you must ask questions* to be sure the "safe bets" are truly that. Don't be afraid to repeatedly ask the waiter or chef how the food is prepared, if there are separate gluten-free prep facilities, or if that thing in your salad that looks like a crouton is really a crouton! Communicate what your needs are, and nine times out of ten they will be more than happy to accommodate.

That's really the one word that encapsulates gluten-free living: accommodation. You have to give a little here and take a little there, but in the end the food you can eat will be delicious, nutritious, and safe. All this info is just the tip of the iceberg, meant to give you a jumping-off point. Read the studies, talk to your doctors and friends, find other people with celiac disease, and get informed. Information is your strongest ally, and more and more is coming out each day. Use it to give yourself the best, and tastiest, life you can!

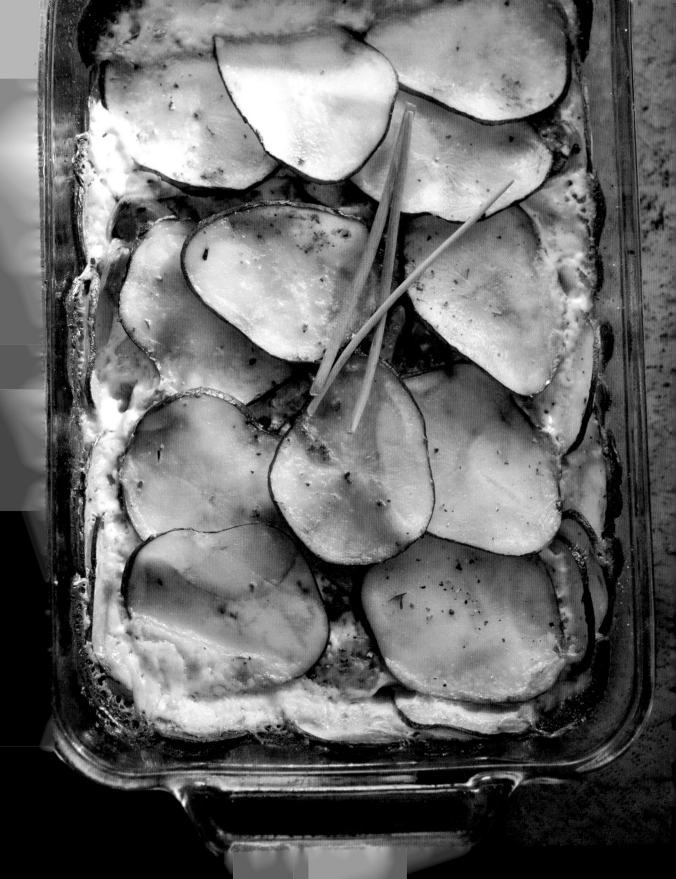

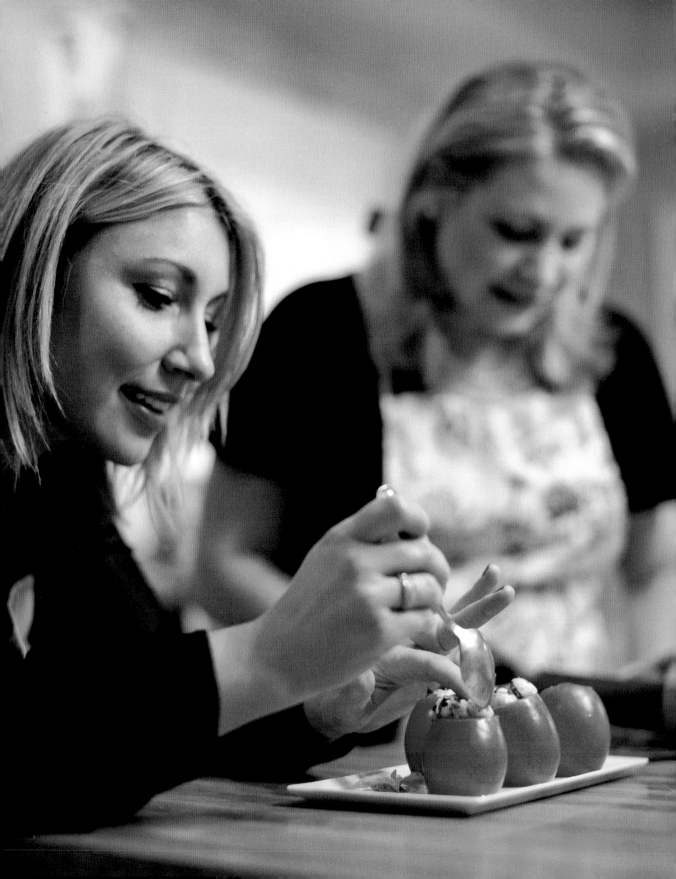

appetizers

Of the two of us, Jilly is definitely the entertainer these days. She loves spending the better part of the day preparing scrumptious little appetizers to thrill her guests. Meanwhile, Jessie spends the better part of *her* day trying to keep her older son from eating the scrumptious little appetizers before his auntie Jilly gets to serve them. And so it goes in our house, anyway!

Since some people have the time to create mini masterpieces and some people don't, we have chosen to include a few of both kinds of appetizers here. None of them literally take half of a day, of course, but some do take a few hours! The time is certainly well spent, though, we are sure you'll agree.

avocado *and* crab cocktail

INGREDIENTS

2 large ripe Hass avocados

1½ lemons

Salt and black pepper to taste

8 ounces white crabmeat, picked through for shells, or shrimp, cooked and coarsely chopped

2 tablespoons mayonnaise

2½ teaspoons Dijon mustard

2 teaspoons Tabasco sauce, preferably green

2 tablespoons finely chopped mix of fresh herbs, such as dill, chives, and tarragon

2 handfuls arugula or watercress (or any peppery lettuce)

Blue or yellow corn tortilla chips, for serving

Who knew that avocados, cut lengthwise, made such great little bowls for filling? This is an impressive appetizer to serve at your next dinner party. For something so beautiful and elegant, they are surprisingly easy to make. As with many mayonnaise-based appetizers, you may want to add a little more or a little less mayonnaise, depending on your preference. Also, feel free to use any mix of fresh herbs below. Serve with a few blue or yellow corn chips on the side to scoop up all this deliciousness. Enjoy.

SERVES 4

STEPS

❶ Cut the avocados in half lengthwise and remove the pit.

❷ Squeeze the juice of the half lemon into a small bowl. With a pastry brush, brush all sides of the avocado halves with the lemon juice, to prevent browning. Season with a bit of salt and pepper.

❸ In a medium-size bowl, combine the crabmeat (or shrimp if substituting), mayonnaise, Dijon mustard, and Tabasco and stir gently to mix well.

❹ Add the fresh herbs, juice from the whole lemon (being careful not to include any seeds), and salt and pepper, and mix well.

❺ Distribute the mixture evenly among the 4 avocado halves.

❻ Place the avocado halves on serving plates, garnish with the lettuce, and serve with tortilla chips on the side.

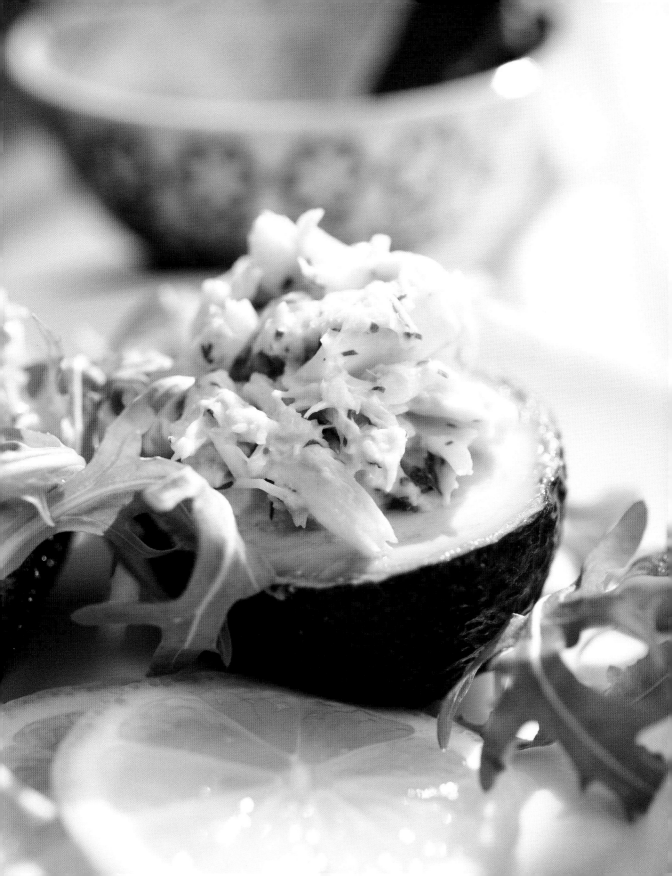

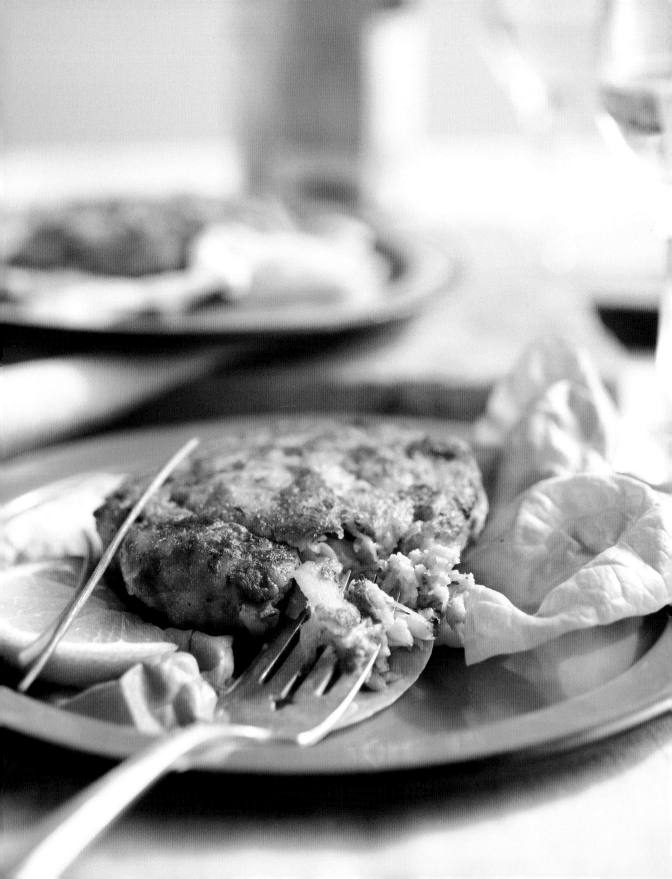

plain jane crab cakes

INGREDIENTS

4 slices gluten-free bread

2 teaspoons olive oil, plus 2 to 4 tablespoons oil for frying

¼ cup chopped chives

¼ cup minced celery

¼ cup minced yellow onion

3 tablespoons finely chopped red bell pepper

2 teaspoons finely chopped fresh parsley

½ teaspoon cayenne pepper

½ teaspoon salt

½ teaspoon dry mustard

1 large egg

¼ cup mayonnaise

½ teaspoon lemon juice

1 pound lump crabmeat, picked through for shells

Tapioca flour, for dusting

We love how crab cakes mix the feel of upscale seafood with the full-bodied pleasure of down-home comfort food. It's no wonder they're among the first to go every time we throw a party! You can make the patties well in advance and fry them up ten to fifteen minutes before everyone arrives. Some people like to complement the taste of crab cakes with a sauce or dip, but we think that serving them plain really brings out the taste of the crabmeat. Feel free to dress them up, though, if you prefer. The formula below makes crab cakes that hit the sweet spot in terms of consistency: moist but crumbly, not too wet and not too dry.

MAKES 8 CAKES

STEPS

❶ Using a food processor, grind the bread pieces into fine crumbs. You should have approximately 2 cups of bread crumbs for this recipe. Set aside.

❷ In a small skillet over medium heat, heat 2 teaspoons of the olive oil. Add the chives, celery, onion, red bell pepper, and parsley and sauté until tender, about 3 minutes.

❸ In a medium-size bowl, toss the bread crumbs with the sautéed vegetables, the cayenne, salt, and mustard until evenly incorporated. Set aside.

❹ In a separate bowl, beat the egg with a wire whisk. Next, whisk in the mayonnaise and lemon juice.

❺ Gently fold the mayonnaise mixture into the bread crumb mixture. Add the crabmeat and mix gently, making sure the crab is evenly distributed throughout.

❻ Divide the mixture into 8 portions and shape each portion into a patty. Lightly coat each patty with the tapioca flour. This will help bind the patties for frying. Place the patties on a cookie sheet, cover with plastic wrap, and refrigerate for at least 30 minutes.

❼ In a large skillet and using as much or as little oil as necessary, fry the crab cakes over medium heat for 2 to 4 minutes on each side. The outside of the cakes should brown and become crispy. Serve alone or with your choice of sauce.

grilled tuna salad *with* capers *and* dill

1½ pounds tuna steaks, each
    1¼ inches thick

Olive oil

Salt and black pepper to taste

½ cup mayonnaise

¼ cup (2 ounces) capers,
    drained

1 tablespoon lemon juice

1½ teaspoons chopped fresh
    dill or ¾ teaspoon dried dill

This tuna dish is surprisingly versatile: it can be served as an appetizer with gluten-free chips or crackers, as the filling for a chunky tuna salad sandwich, or on a crisp bed of greens as a tuna salad! The dill especially adds a nice flavor to this dish. We prefer fresh dill, but dried dill will also do the trick. The tuna steaks will cook just as well on an indoor grill as on an outdoor one. Just remember to reduce your cooking time to compensate for the two-sided indoor version. This is a classic lunch or appetizer with lots of options *and* lots of flavor…perfect!

SERVES 6 TO 8 AS AN APPETIZER

STEPS

❶ Preheat the grill.

❷ Brush the tuna steaks on both sides with olive oil. Season on both sides with salt and pepper.

❸ Grill until the fish is browned on the outside but pink on the inside, about 6 to 8 minutes on each side if preparing on an outdoor grill. If using a two-sided (contact) indoor grill, reduce the cooking time to 3 to 5 minutes. Set the cooked fish aside to cool.

❹ Once the fish is cool, chop roughly into chunks.

❺ In a medium-size bowl, combine the mayonnaise, capers, lemon juice, and dill and stir to mix well. Gently incorporate the tuna into the mixture.

❻ Re-season with salt and pepper to your desired preference. Remember that capers are usually salty, so make sure you sample the mixture before adding more salt.

❼ Chill for at least a half hour to allow flavors to meld before serving.

coconut-lime shrimp
and artichoke skewers

INGREDIENTS

½ cup coconut milk, light if preferred

Juice and grated zest of 1 lime

2 teaspoons Emeril's Fish Rub or Original Essence Seasoning, or fish rub or Cajun seasoning of your choice

Salt and black pepper to taste

12 large shrimp, rinsed, peeled, and deveined

1 can (14 ounces) artichoke hearts, drained well (about 1 cup)

These tasty little skewers have become a summer staple in our homes. They hit all the major selling points: healthy, light, tasty, but also very quick to put together. Remember, you don't want to marinate the shrimp for more than 15 minutes. Any longer and the lime juice will start to cook the shrimp and make them tough when grilled. The skewers grill in 5 minutes flat and taste great on either an outdoor grill or your favorite indoor variety. We recommend serving them as an appetizer or trying them on top of your favorite salad for a more filling meal. The recipe below was developed to serve two, so it's easy to double, depending on the number of guests you have. Your guests will love how delicious they are, and you'll love how easy they are to prepare.

SERVES 2 (12 SHRIMP WILL MAKE 4 SKEWERS)

STEPS

❶ In a medium-size bowl, combine the coconut milk, half the lime juice, the lime zest, the Fish Rub or Essence Seasoning, and a bit of salt and pepper. Stir well. Add the shrimp and stir to coat.

❷ Cover with cling film and chill in the refrigerator for no longer than 15 minutes.

❸ Meanwhile, preheat the grill and have ready 4 metal or wooden skewers, soaking wooden skewers in water before using them.

❹ Take the bowl out of the refrigerator and drain the shrimp, discarding the marinade.

❺ Assemble the skewers, following an alternating pattern of shrimp and artichoke hearts. There should be 3 shrimp and 2 artichoke hearts per skewer.

❻ Place on the hot grill and cook 2½ minutes on each side or until cooked through.

❼ Sprinkle the shrimp with the remaining lime juice and serve.

stuffed roma tomatoes

8 fresh, ripe Roma tomatoes

1 pound fresh mozzarella, either cubed or torn into bite-size piece (about 2 cups)

4 heaping tablespoons finely chopped fresh basil

1 teaspoon dried oregano or 2 teaspoons finely chopped fresh oregano

2 tablespoons extra virgin olive oil

4 teaspoons balsamic vinegar

Salt and black pepper to taste

These hollowed-out and stuffed Roma tomatoes not only embody one of history's most timeless flavor combinations; they also make cute and delicious appetizers. We consider them our quirky appetizer version of a Caprese salad, balancing fresh basil and soft, fresh, creamy mozzarella with the bright acid of the tomato. They're simply delicious! We love the way these little guys stand up on their own, too. Just be sure not to trim too much off the bottoms or else the stuffing will not stay in.

Depending on the size of the Roma tomatoes you have available, you might end up with some stuffing left over. All the better to taste test it straight away with a fork or some gluten-free crackers. After all that work stuffing each individual tomato, you deserve it!

SERVES 8

STEPS

1 For each tomato, cut off the first ¼ to ½ inch of the top and bottom so the tomato stands up on its own.

2 Using a grapefruit spoon or melon baller, carefully hollow out each tomato, making sure not to poke a hole through the bottom.

3 In a medium-size bowl, combine the remaining ingredients and toss gently until evenly distributed.

4 Using a teaspoon, stuff the mozzarella mixture into the hollowed-out tomatoes. Any extra stuffing can be refrigerated and used or eaten within a day or two.

5 Chill for at least 15 minutes before serving.

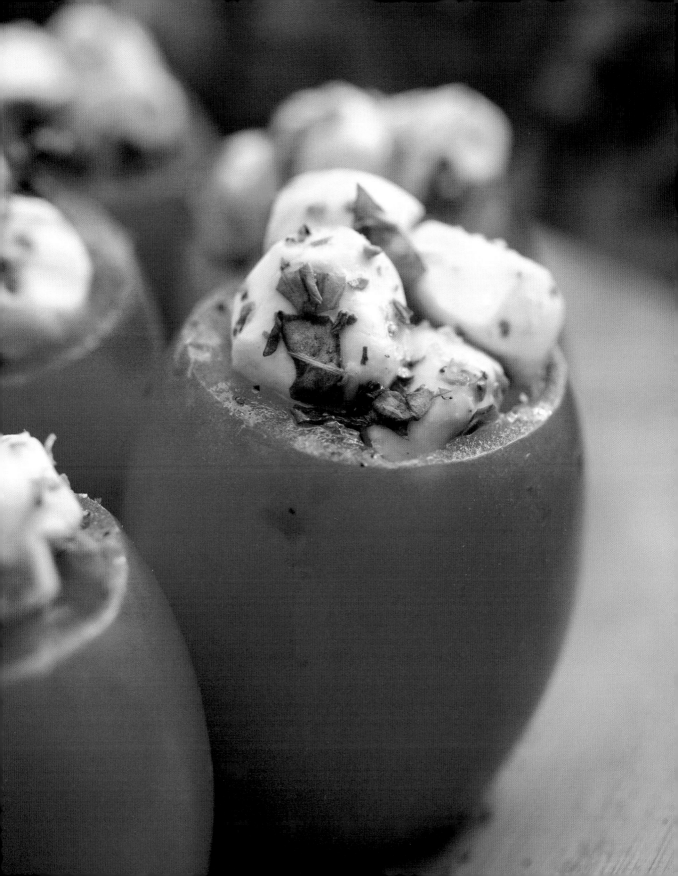

jilly *and* jude's basil pesto dip *with* homemade crackers

INGREDIENTS

crackers

2 cups (plus extra for dusting) gluten-free all-purpose flour blend (we've used Arrowhead Mills Gluten Free All Purpose Baking Mix)

½ cup water

¼ cup olive oil

3 tablespoons freshly grated Parmesan cheese

1 tablespoon Italian seasoning blend

½ teaspoon salt

¼ teaspoon black pepper

¼ teaspoon garlic powder

pesto

8 ounces cream cheese, low-fat if preferred, in one block

2 large fresh, ripe tomatoes (vine or beefsteak)

2 large handfuls fresh basil leaves, rinsed and patted dry

½ teaspoon minced garlic (roughly 1 clove)

¼ cup freshly grated Parmesan cheese

¼ cup extra virgin olive oil

Salt and black pepper to taste

When we were younger, going to our auntie Barbara's house was a childhood highlight. She was a wonderful cook, like many people in our family, and always had a delightful spread no matter who came to visit. Auntie Barbara and her daughter, Lisel, would create the magic in the kitchen while the rest of us were shooed away or steered in the direction of the pool to keep us occupied. One year, though, Cousin Lisel invited Jilly in and introduced her to the art of making this fresh pesto dip, chock full of fresh herbs, tomatoes, and yummy cream cheese. Just one taste reminds Jilly of summer gatherings at Auntie Barbara's house, creating wonderful memories with all our family. Now, all these years later, Auntie Jilly makes the pesto dip whenever she visits, with the help of Jessie's son Jude. Jude helps his aunt by picking the basil leaves from Jessie's garden and then, of course, pressing all the buttons on the blender. He is extremely instrumental in mixing up all the mouthwatering ingredients for the crackers, too!

SERVES 6 TO 10

STEPS

crackers

1 Preheat the oven to 350°F.

2 In a medium-size bowl, mix all the ingredients together to make a dough.

3 Form the dough into a ball, and divide it into 2 smaller balls.

4 Generously dust a work surface and rolling pin with more flour blend.

5 Gently roll out each ball of dough as thinly as possible without letting it crumble into pieces.

6 With either a cookie cutter or pizza cutter, cut the dough into pieces. As long as the thickness of the dough is pretty uniform, you can make the crackers in any shape you like.

7 Transfer the shapes to baking trays and bake for 15 to 20 minutes, or until golden brown.

8 Allow to cool on the baking trays before transferring. The crackers will crisp as they cool. Store any leftovers in an airtight container.

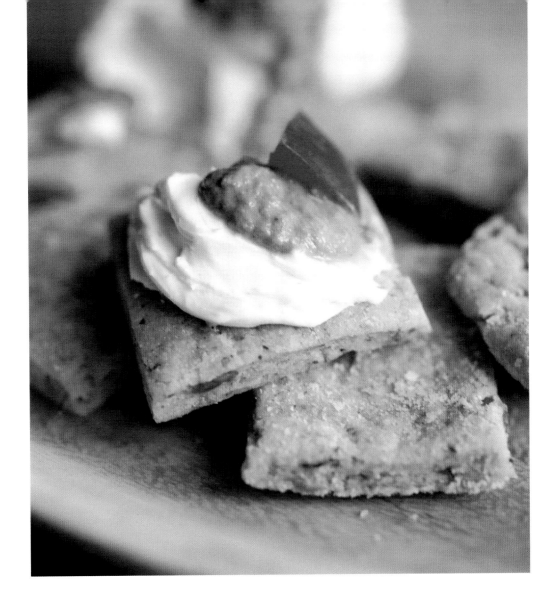

pesto

1 Unwrap the cream cheese, place on a serving plate or platter, and allow to come to room temperature.

2 Cut one of the tomatoes crosswise in half. Seed and chop one of the halves and set aside.

3 Coarsely chop the remaining tomatoes and place in a blender or food processor. Add the basil, garlic, Parmesan cheese, extra virgin olive oil, and a good pinch of salt and pepper. Blend until smooth.

4 Taste and adjust the seasoning with salt and pepper as desired.

5 Pour the pesto over the cream cheese block on the serving platter.

6 Sprinkle the reserved chopped tomato on top of the pesto and cream cheese.

7 Serve immediately, with the homemade gluten-free crackers.

zucchini *and* polenta fritters

INGREDIENTS

- 3 small to medium-size zucchini, rinsed well, ends chopped off and discarded
- ¾ cup gluten-free all-purpose flour blend (we've used Arrowhead Mills Gluten Free All Purpose Baking Mix)
- 2 medium-size eggs, beaten
- ⅓ cup milk, any % fat you prefer
- ½ cup cornmeal or polenta, or more as needed
- 2½ tablespoons fresh lemon thyme or regular thyme leaves
- Pinch of crushed red pepper flakes
- Salt and black pepper to taste
- 1½ tablespoons vegetable oil
- 1 lemon, sliced into wedges

Jilly came up with this recipe one summer in London after a very successful attempt at growing zucchini in her new vegetable garden—perhaps too successful. She soon had an overabundance of veggies and had to find something to do with all that zucchini! It was grilled, it was chopped and added to homemade pasta sauces, and eventually it was fried. And here is where she struck gold.

These tasty fritters are a great addition to any antipasto. You can also make a meal out of them, by simply serving alongside some good-quality Italian olives, your favorite cheeses, marinated artichoke hearts, and a big glass of wine. They are wonderful served with some of the homemade pesto in our Jilly and Jude's Basil Pesto Dip recipe (page 28). You can fry them in any size you like. Just make sure to use a nonstick skillet to avoid overly oily fritters. Try passing a small version of these at your next cocktail party!

MAKES ROUGHLY 12 TO 14 FRITTERS

STEPS

❶ Grate the zucchini with a hand-held grater or in a food processor.

❷ Place the grated zucchini in a bowl lined with paper towels. Place more paper towels over the zucchini and press down to draw out any excess liquid. After absorbing as much liquid as possible, set the zucchini aside.

❸ Sift the flour blend into a large bowl and make a well in the center, using your hands.

❹ Add the eggs to the well and gradually draw in the flour, using your hands or a wooden spoon.

❺ Slowly add the milk and ½ cup of the cornmeal or polenta to the mixture, stirring constantly until a thick batter forms.

❻ Add the drained grated zucchini, thyme, crushed red pepper flakes, and a bit of salt and pepper to the batter and mix well. If the mixture seems too moist, add a bit more cornmeal or polenta and stir.

7 Heat the oil in a large skillet over medium heat.

8 Once the oil is hot, spoon the fritter mixture into the pan by heaping tablespoonfuls and cook until golden brown on each side, about 3 to 4 minutes per side, flipping once during cooking. Once flipped, press down gently with the spatula to help the fritters cook faster.

9 Remove the fritters carefully with the spatula and place on a paper towel–lined plate to absorb any excess oil.

10 Repeat steps 8 and 9 until all the batter has been used.

11 Before serving, season with a bit more salt and pepper and a squeeze of lemon juice while still warm.

fresh tuna *and* butter lettuce wraps *with* shaved jalapeño *and* basil oil

INGREDIENTS

wraps

1 recipe Ponzu (recipe follows)

16 (½-ounce) slices sushi-grade yellowfin tuna, sliced ¼ inch thick

16 large butter lettuce leaves

16 paper-thin slices fresh jalapeño

Spicy chili garlic sauce, for garnish (recommended: Sriracha)

16 sprigs cilantro

Basil Oil (recipe follows)

ponzu

1 cup tamari or gluten-free soy sauce

½ cup sugar

2 inches fresh ginger, cut into ⅛-inch slices

2 lemons, juiced

2 oranges, juiced

basil oil

1 cup (loosely packed) basil leaves

½ cup olive oil

We usually beg and plead with our dad to make us these beautiful tuna lettuce wraps, which are nothing short of mini parcels full of deliciousness! He is more than happy to oblige, more so if he's had a successful day out fishing on his boat. Filled with the refreshing tang from the citrus and Ponzu sauce, followed by a slight heat from the shaved jalapeños and Sriracha chili garlic sauce, they really are a flavor-packed bit. Light, clean, and refreshing. Everyone will enjoy these.

MAKES 4 LARGE APPETIZERS

STEPS

wraps

❶ Pour ¼ cup of the Ponzu onto a large dinner plate. Carefully lay the slices of tuna in the sauce. Marinate for 1 minute. Turn the tuna over and marinate it for another minute.

❷ Arrange the lettuce leaves on 4 dinner plates, placing 4 leaves on each plate to make a four-leaf-clover pattern. Place 1 slice of tuna on top of each lettuce leaf.

❸ Pour ½ teaspoon of the Ponzu over each slice.

❹ Place 1 slice of jalapeño on top of each piece of tuna, followed by a dot of the Sriracha and a sprig of cilantro.

❺ Drizzle each plate with a small amount of the Basil Oil and serve.

ponzu

❶ Combine all the ingredients in a nonreactive saucepan and bring to a simmer. Stir until the sugar is dissolved, about 5 minutes. Remove from the heat and allow to cool before using.

❷ Keep covered in the refrigerator for up to 2 months.

basil oil

❶ Bring 2 cups of water to a boil in a small saucepan. Submerge the basil leaves in the water for 10 seconds, or until completely wilted. Drain.

❷ Shock under cold running water. Blot the leaves on a paper towel to dry them. Place them in a blender with the olive oil and puree for 15 seconds or until completely pureed. Reserve the oil in a squeeze bottle. Will keep for 1 week refrigerated.

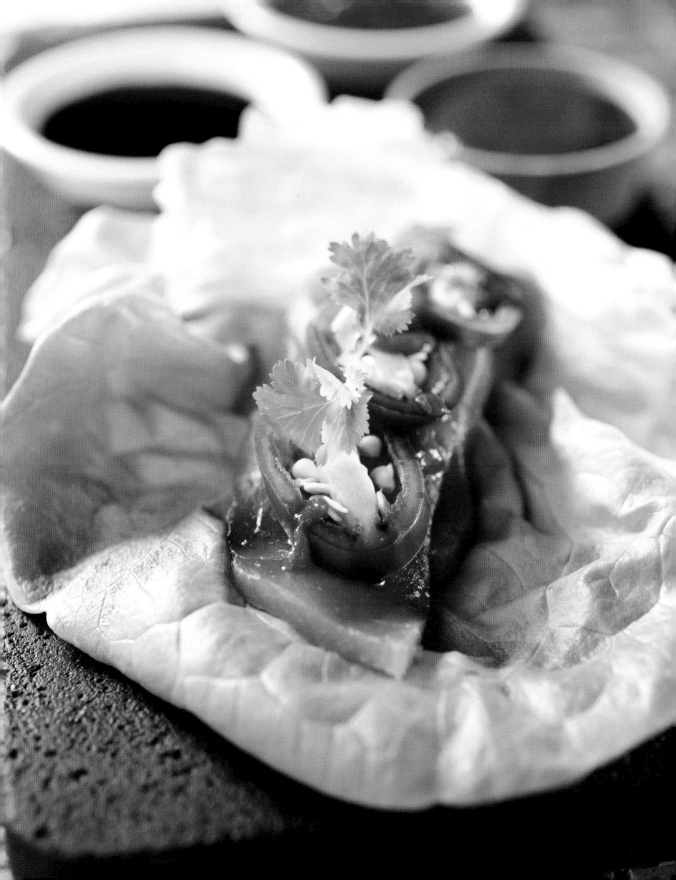

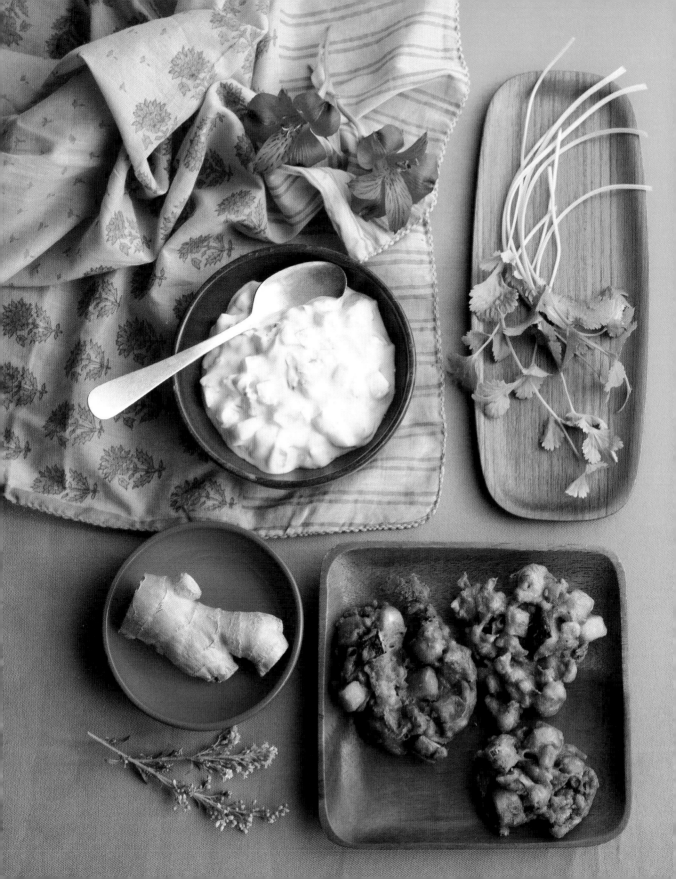

indian vegetable pakoras
with cucumber raita

INGREDIENTS

batter

1½ cups chickpea flour (aka gram or garbanzo flour)

1 teaspoon ground cumin

2 teaspoons garam masala

1 teaspoon hot curry or Madras curry powder

2½ teaspoons caraway seeds

Generous pinch of salt

1 teaspoon finely chopped fresh ginger

3 tablespoons finely chopped fresh cilantro

¾ to 1 cup warm water, as needed

vegetables

½ small potato, peeled and cut into small bite-size cubes

½ small yellow onion, chopped

Salt

Vegetable oil for frying (amount depends on the pan you're using to fry—see step 3)

½ cup cauliflower florets, cut into bite-size pieces

½ small zucchini, cut into bite-size pieces

1 to 2 red or green chilies, seeded, deveined, and finely chopped

Living in London for so long, Jilly now insists on two things in life: a year-round tan and delicious Indian food at least twice a week! This recipe has all the tastes, smells, and colors she adores and seeks out in authentic Indian food. It truly does awaken all the senses. All the ingredients and frying may frighten even the most seasoned of cooks, but we assure you that these incredible pakoras are worth the effort. They are a special treat for your guests, who will certainly taste the effort and love that went into making them. As a great twist, you can substitute paneer, a delicious Indian curd cheese, for the potato. Just dice it and put it into the batter. Yum! Although Jilly does get homesick for the US from time to time, listening to her Indian girlfriends talk about their pakora recipes makes her feel right at home. Whether you're from New Orleans, London, or Mumbai, everyone thinks their momma's recipe is the best!

A raita is a yogurt-based condiment, served alongside most Indian and Pakistani food, that is meant to cool and ease the heat of some dishes. The possibilities of what you can put in a raita are endless. In some regions, they are a main dish in themselves, served with nothing more than naan bread. Normally, you would be served a homemade chutney, mango perhaps, alongside fried pakoras or bharjis. We love the refreshing mint and cooling cucumber in this version. It lightens and balances the heaviness of the substantial pakoras. Feel free to experiment with what you like.

MAKES ABOUT 15 PAKORAS

STEPS

batter

1 In a large bowl, combine the flour, cumin, garam masala, curry powder, caraway seeds, and salt and stir to mix thoroughly.

2 Stir in the ginger and cilantro.

3 Slowly add the water, ¼ cup at a time, until a batter starts to form. A thicker batter is easier to fry; a thinner batter is a bit harder.

(recipe continues)

raita

1 cup full-fat plain yogurt (don't use light or fat-free here)

2 tablespoons water

½ cup peeled, seeded, and chopped English cucumber

1½ teaspoons finely chopped fresh mint

¾ teaspoon granulated sugar

½ teaspoon ground coriander

⅛ teaspoon ground cumin

Pinch of salt

❹ Mix the batter for 1 to 2 minutes, using a fork to remove most lumps and to achieve as smooth a consistency as possible.

❺ Cover the bowl loosely with a piece of paper towel and leave to rest for 30 minutes.

Prepare the vegetables while the batter rests.

vegetables

❶ Place the potatoes in a small bowl of cold salted water and let sit for 15 minutes. Drain and pat dry. Set aside.

❷ Toss the onion with a generous pinch of salt in another small bowl. Set aside for 15 minutes as well. Drain and pat dry. Set aside.

❸ Using either a deep fryer or a heavy pan such as a deep cast-iron skillet, heat the oil to 350°F on medium to low heat. (You need a depth of at least 2 inches with several inches of space above the oil to fry safely and avoid having it bubble over.)

❹ Just before you are ready to fry, add all the vegetables to the batter and mix well.

❺ Start adding the batter, 2 to 3 ladlefuls at a time to avoid overcrowding. (We found using a small ladle to pour the batter into the oil very helpful. Think golf ball–size as opposed to tennis ball–size. We also used a spider spoon, a stir-fry cooking utensil that proved perfect for flipping the fritters.) Fry for 2 to 3 minutes or until golden brown on each side.

❻ Let cool on a baker's rack or a paper towel–lined plate to absorb excess oil.

❼ Serve warm with the raita. (If you need to reheat the pakoras, simply place on a baking sheet in a 350°F oven for 5 minutes, or until crisp again.)

raita

❶ In a small bowl combine the yogurt and water and stir well with a fork.

❷ Add all the remaining ingredients and stir well.

❸ Transfer to a serving bowl and serve with the pakoras.

sweet 'n' sticky chicken wingettes

INGREDIENTS

8 small chicken wingettes or drumsticks

2 tablespoons gluten-free soy sauce or tamari

2 tablespoons honey

1 tablespoon sunflower or vegetable oil

1 tablespoon Dijon or Creole mustard

1 teaspoon tomato sauce

¼ teaspoon grated fresh ginger

Generous pinch of crushed red pepper flakes

Pinch of salt

2 green onions, thinly sliced, for garnish

These tasty little wingettes always seem to be a crowd pleaser at our get-togethers. And luckily for you intrepid hosts, they are a cinch to prepare. We have found these work better using "wingettes," or the smaller version of a chicken drumstick. If you can't find them at your local grocery store, try to use the smallest drumstick you can find. These work equally well cooked on an outdoor grill or baked in the oven. The choice is yours. These are Jessie's son Jude's favorite party snacks, especially because he can use his hands to eat them! Sticky and sweet, tangy and tasty, these little wingettes will be sure to please.

MAKES 8 WINGETTES

STEPS

❶ With a sharp knife, score each drumstick or wingette three times to allow the marinade to penetrate, and place in a medium bowl.

❷ In a small bowl, combine the soy sauce or tamari, honey, oil, mustard, tomato sauce, ginger, red pepper flakes, and salt and mix well.

❸ Pour this mixture over the chicken, making sure the wingettes are evenly coated.

❹ Cover with cling film and place in the refrigerator to marinate for at least 30 minutes, but no longer than 24 hours.

❺ Before cooking, allow the chicken to come to room temperature to make sure the meat will be tender and juicy when cooked, not tough and chewy.

❻ Preheat the oven to 375°F.

❼ Spray a baking tray with a nonstick olive oil spray.

❽ Place the wingettes on the prepared baking tray and bake for 30 to 35 minutes, depending on size, until cooked fully through. Turn once during cooking.

❾ Transfer to a serving platter and garnish with the sliced green onions.

mini goat cheese *and* fig pizzas

INGREDIENTS

pizza

1⅓ cups milk, any % fat you prefer

2 teaspoons olive oil

2 teaspoons red wine or apple cider vinegar

1 teaspoon granulated sugar

2⅓ cups gluten-free all-purpose flour blend (we've used Arrowhead Mills Gluten Free All Purpose Baking Mix), plus extra for dusting

⅓ cup coarse-ground yellow cornmeal, plus extra

2 heaping teaspoons xanthan gum

½ teaspoon salt

½ teaspoon garlic salt

8 ounces goat cheese (chèvre), best quality possible

8 fresh figs, any variety, stems removed, cut into roughly 8 to 10 lengthwise slices per fig, depending on size, or fig preserves, enough to cover tops of pizzas

Red Onion Chutney (recipe follows)

Fresh chives, finely chopped, for garnish (optional)

red onion chutney

2½ tablespoons olive oil

2 medium-size red onions, halved crosswise, then halved again lengthwise and very thinly sliced (about 2 cups)

Salt and black pepper to taste

1 tablespoon balsamic vinegar

1 tablespoon (packed) light brown sugar

These may seem a bit daunting to make, but rest assured, you can make and cook the pizza crusts in advance so all you're left with is a quick assembly of the remaining delicious bits. The pizza crust recipe is purposefully yeast free. It works and tastes great without it and is perfect for individuals who suffer from yeast sensitivity. The dough is incredibly versatile: if you have any left over, roll it out, sprinkle it with a bit of garlic salt or Parmesan cheese, and bake it off as breadsticks or a savory flatbread. The possibilities are endless, but always delicious. As for the tempting mini pizzas, who doesn't love the combination of sweet goat cheese and syrupy figs? Add the tanginess of the red onion chutney and you have a winning recipe.

Keep in mind that as scrumptious as figs are, they unfortunately do not transport well and aren't always available year round. So you can always substitute a good-quality fig preserve, like St. Dalfour Royal Fig Preserves, for the fresh variety. Just spoon a bit of the preserves on top of the onion chutney.

Try these out as passed hors d'oeuvres at your next dinner party and get ready for the compliment train. Everyone will be on board for these!

MAKES 14 TO 16 PIZZAS

STEPS

pizza

❶ Preheat the oven to 400°F.

❷ In a small bowl, combine the milk, olive oil, vinegar, and sugar and stir well until the sugar is dissolved. Set aside.

❸ In a medium-size bowl, combine the 2⅓ cups flour blend, ⅓ cup cornmeal, the xanthan gum, and the salts.

❹ Add the wet ingredients to the dry ingredients and stir with a fork until well incorporated and a dough forms.

❺ Divide the dough in half to make it easier to work with. Place one of the dough halves on a surface that's well floured with flour blend, or on a piece of parchment paper, and sprinkle generously all over with some cornmeal. This makes it easier to roll out.

(recipe continues)

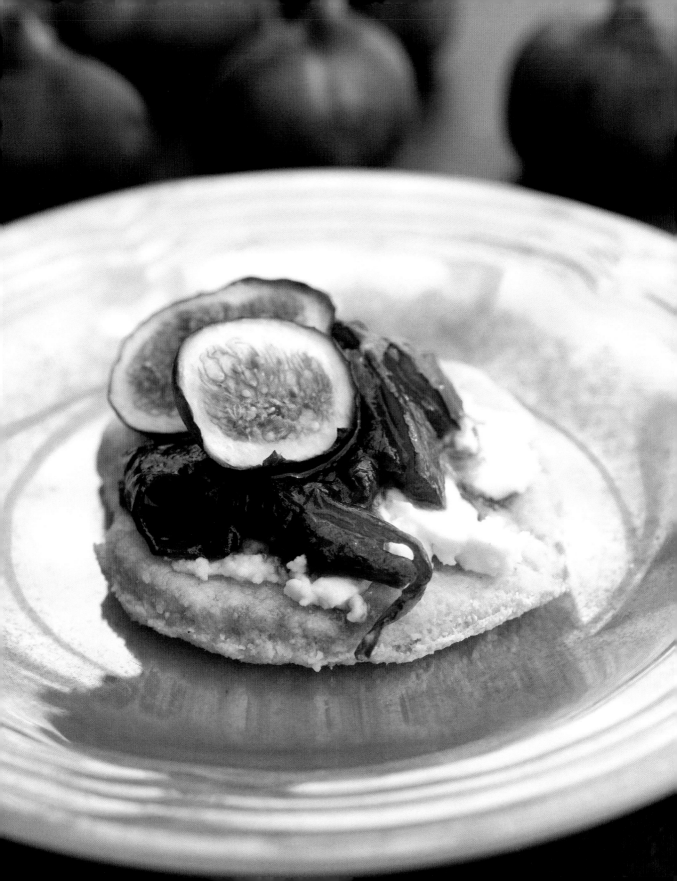

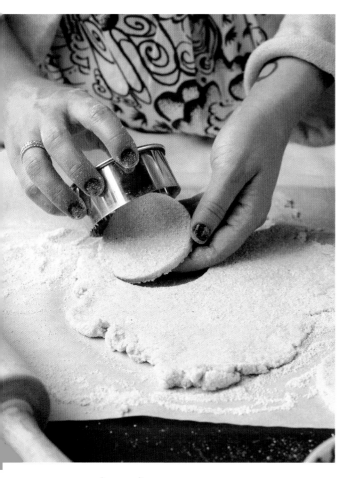

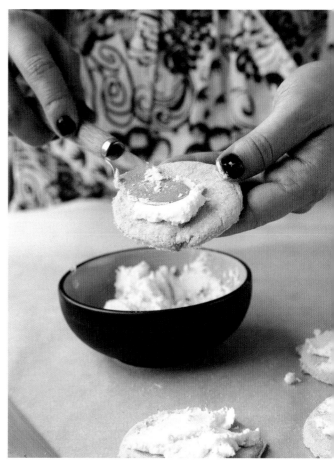

6 With a floured rolling pin, roll the dough out as thinly and evenly as possible without it cracking, anywhere between ¼ and ⅛ inch thick. If the dough gets too sticky to handle, simply sprinkle with a bit more cornmeal.

7 Using a circular cookie cutter with a 3-inch diameter, cut out as many circles as possible, making sure both sides of the circles are well coated with the cornmeal (see photo). Lay them 1 inch apart on baking trays.

8 Add any remaining dough scraps to the other half of the dough that has been set aside and repeat steps 6 to 8 until all the dough has been used. Any remaining scraps can be baked off as breadsticks or discarded.

9 Bake the pizza crust circles for 10 to 12 minutes, or until slightly golden brown.

10 Remove the baking trays from the oven and reduce the oven temperature to 375°F. Allow the pizza crusts to cool directly on the trays before assembling.

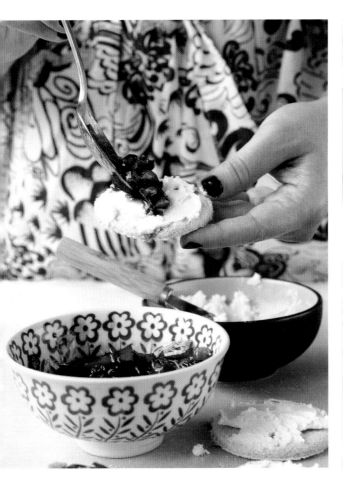
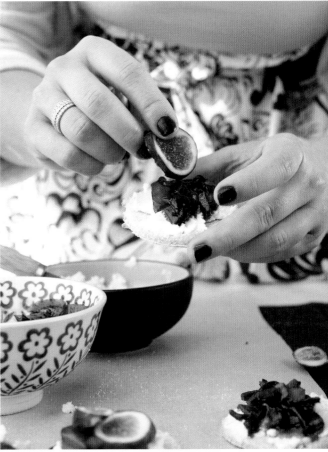

⑪ Spoon about a tablespoon of goat cheese on each cooled crust and spread it out as evenly as possible (see photo).

⑫ Spoon a small amount of the Red Onion Chutney on top of the cheese, trying to distribute the mixture as evenly as possible among the crusts (see photo).

⑬ Place 2 slices of fig on top of each pizza (see photo) and bake for 4 to 5 minutes, or until the figs start to wilt slightly and the cheese is warmed through. If you are using a fig preserve, gently spoon a small amount of the preserve on top of the chutney.

⑭ Remove from the oven, place on a serving platter, garnish with a sprinkle of the finely chopped chives, if desired, and serve warm.

red onion chutney

❶ In a small saucepan over medium-low heat, heat the olive oil. Add the onion and sauté with a bit of salt and pepper until softened, about 6 minutes.

❷ Add the balsamic vinegar and brown sugar and cook another 4 to 6 minutes, stirring constantly. The mixture will start to have a syrupy consistency.

❸ Turn off the heat and set the chutney aside in the pan to cool.

thai turkey meatballs *with* homemade thai sweet chili dipping sauce

INGREDIENTS

meatballs

2½ tablespoons nuoc mam (Thai fish sauce)

1 small stalk fresh lemongrass, finely chopped, with any discolored outer leaves discarded

1 small red chili, seeded, deveined, and finely chopped

1 pound lean ground turkey

3 green onions, finely chopped

2 tablespoons chopped fresh cilantro

1 heaping tablespoon chopped fresh mint, plus extra for garnish

1 heaping tablespoon chopped fresh Thai basil, plus extra for garnish

1 tablespoon tapioca flour or cornstarch, plus extra for dusting hands

Pinch of granulated sugar

Pinch of salt

1½ teaspoons vegetable or sunflower oil

Thai Sweet Chili Dipping Sauce (recipe follows), for serving (optional)

We can't tell you how delicious and addictive these flavor-packed meatballs are…you and your guests won't be able to eat just one! The chili offers just the right touch of heat, yet your palette is instantly cooled by the refreshing taste of mint and basil. You might have eaten a similar version of this dish at your favorite Thai restaurant, where the meatballs are usually served with a coconut sauce and perhaps with noodles. Traditionally, they are rolled in either bread or panko crumbs, but we've used tapioca flour to make these tasty Thai delights happily gluten-free. You can serve them warm or cold, but they are particularly excellent served alongside a small ramekin of Thai sweet chili dipping sauce. You can use a store-bought variety or try the homemade version we've included, if you're up to it. The spicy, sweet, and tangy sauce tastes good on just about anything! You can use fresh chilies, as we have done or, if it's easier, you can substitute ½ to 1 tablespoon of crushed red pepper flakes. Depending on your palate, you may find yourself wanting it a bit sweeter or spicier. Simply add more sugar or chili to suit your taste buds. Just remember that when working with raw chilies, the heat is actually in the membrane and seeds, so proceed accordingly. And *always* wash your hands or wear latex gloves when handling chilies (we speak from personal experience—why *did* I rub my eye?!). This recipe also makes a great housewarming gift: simply store it in a sterile mason jar or decorative airtight container, pop a bow on, and voilà. The sauce keeps fabulously well in the refrigerator for months on end, and if anything, it just gets more flavorful with age, just like a good red wine.

You'll be surprised how many guests will end up asking you for the recipe. Even Jessie's three-year-old son, Jude, came for seconds…and thirds!

Obviously these are wonderful as an appetizer, but for a more filling meal, you can serve with a steaming bowl of spicy rice noodles and your favorite steamed veggies. Enjoy!

MAKES ROUGHLY 20 GOLF BALL–SIZE MEATBALLS

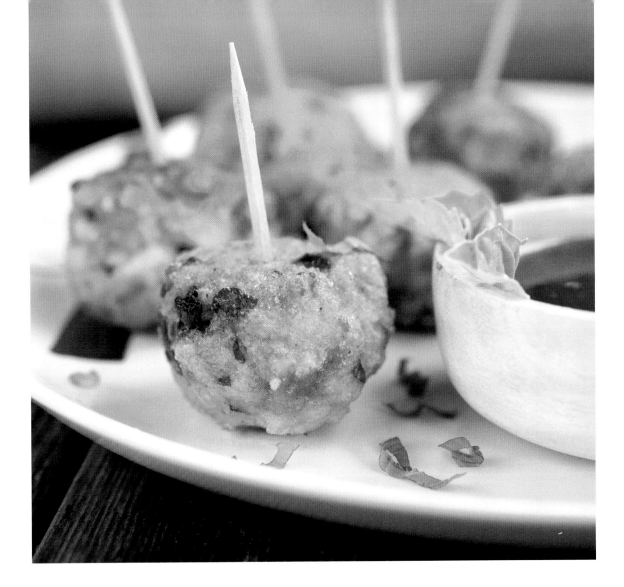

meatballs

1 In a 1-quart or smaller saucepan, gently cook the fish sauce and lemongrass on low heat for 3 to 4 minutes, to soften the lemongrass. Take the saucepan off the heat and allow the mixture to cool slightly.

2 In a medium-size bowl, combine the red chili, ground turkey, green onions, fresh herbs, tapioca flour, sugar, and salt.

3 Add the cooled fish sauce–lemongrass mixture and mix well, using either your hands or a spoon to distribute all the ingredients evenly.

4 Lightly flour your hands and form as many small balls, each about the size of a golf ball, as the mixture allows. You'll need to reflour your hands before rolling each ball.

5 Place the meatballs on a baking tray and chill in the refrigerator for 30 minutes, uncovered.

(recipe continues)

thai sweet chili dipping sauce

MAKES ROUGHLY 1¼ CUPS SAUCE

1 small fresh red jalapeño, seeded and deveined

½ to ¾ cup granulated sugar, depending on sweetness desired

¾ cup plus 2 tablespoons water

¼ cup white or rice wine vinegar

2 tablespoons nuoc mam (Thai fish sauce)

2 cloves garlic, chopped

1½ teaspoons salt

1 tablespoon cornstarch

6 In a large nonstick skillet, heat the oil over medium heat.

7 Once the oil is hot, fry the meatballs until fully cooked, about 15 to 20 minutes. Gently turn the meatballs while frying until they are golden and crispy on all sides.

8 Drain the cooked meatballs on a paper towel–lined plate to absorb any excess oil.

9 Transfer to a serving plate or platter and skewer each meatball with a toothpick.

10 Garnish the plate with the reserved chopped basil and mint and serve along with a small ramekin of Thai Sweet Chili Dipping Sauce.

thai sweet chili dipping sauce

1 Put all the ingredients except the cornstarch and the 2 tablespoons water into a blender and blend until everything is well combined and any jalapeño chunks are pureed.

2 Transfer the mixture to a medium-size nonstick saucepan and bring to a gentle boil over medium-high heat. Boil for 5 minutes, making sure the sauce doesn't foam over. The smell of the vinegar burning off may be a bit strong or pungent; this is perfectly normal.

3 Turn the heat down to low and simmer until the sauce starts to thicken, about 3 to 4 minutes.

4 In a small bowl, dissolve the cornstarch in the 2 tablespoons water.

5 Add this to the sauce in the pan, turn the heat back up to high, and let the sauce bubble slightly for 1 minute, whisking constantly. It should be thickening up.

6 Turn the heat back down to low and taste, adding more sugar, if desired, now before turning off the heat.

7 Allow the sauce to cool completely before serving.

8 If not using immediately, transfer to a sterilized Mason jar or other airtight container and store in the refrigerator.

hot mama's spinach *and* artichoke dip

INGREDIENTS

8 ounces low-fat cream cheese, softened to room temperature

1 cup light sour cream

½ cup freshly grated Parmesan cheese

1 cup grated fontina cheese

½ yellow bell pepper, cored, seeded, and finely chopped

½ red bell pepper, cored, seeded, and finely chopped

1 box (10 ounces) frozen chopped spinach, thawed and drained

3 cloves garlic, minced

1½ teaspoons Emeril's Original Essence Seasoning or Cajun seasoning of your choice

Pinch of cayenne pepper

Black pepper to taste

1 can or jar (14 ounces) artichoke hearts, drained well and chopped

4 green onions, thinly sliced

Please tell us who on Earth doesn't die for spinach and artichoke dip? Seriously, show yourselves! Whenever we were both home in New Orleans, we always tried to go to one of our favorite restaurants, Houston's, where they make the most amazing spinach and artichoke dip, among many other things. It wasn't until recently that we found out that their version is prepared using a béchamel sauce with wheat flour. Oh no! Cue our mission to make a hot little version of this dip, our way, deliciously full of flavor and completely gluten-free. We used fontina cheese as opposed to the customary mozzarella. The nuttiness of the cheese adds a nice dimension to the usual flavors. Serve with vegetable crudités or your favorite gluten-free corn tortilla chips, or Jilly's personal favorite, a cold margarita. This tasty party dip won't last long. Now all you need is the party!

SERVES 8 TO 10

STEPS

❶ Preheat the oven to 350°F.

❷ Place the cream cheese, sour cream, Parmesan, ½ cup of the fontina, and the bell peppers in a large bowl.

❸ Squeeze out any excess liquid from the thawed spinach and add to the bowl.

❹ Add the garlic, Essence Seasoning, cayenne, and a bit of black pepper. Stir vigorously until thoroughly mixed.

❺ Add the chopped artichoke hearts and half of the green onions and stir well.

❻ Spoon the mixture into an 8 × 8–inch baking dish.

❼ Sprinkle the remaining ½ cup fontina cheese evenly over the top and bake for 30 minutes, or until the cheese on top is bubbly and melted.

❽ Garnish with the remaining green onions and serve warm.

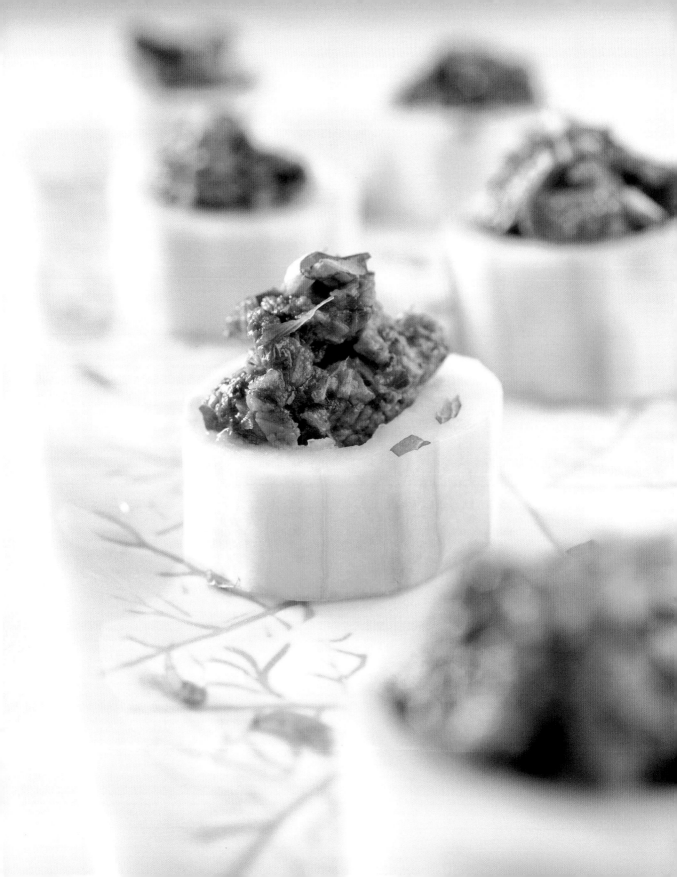

lemongrass *and* chili beef *in* cucumber cups

INGREDIENTS

- 1 stalk fresh lemongrass, finely chopped, with any discolored outer leaves discarded
- 3 cloves garlic, minced
- 1 small red chili pepper, seeded, deveined, and roughly chopped
- 2 tablespoons granulated sugar
- 1 tablespoon nuoc mam (Thai fish sauce)
- 1 tablespoon vegetable or sunflower oil
- 1½ teaspoons gluten-free soy sauce or tamari
- ½ teaspoon toasted sesame oil
- Small handful of fresh basil leaves, finely chopped
- Small handful of fresh mint, finely chopped, plus additional for garnish
- ½ pound flank or skirt steak
- 2 large English cucumbers, seedless if possible

These lil' babies take some preparation, but they are simply packed with delicious Vietnamese flavors—sweet, spicy, crisp, and refreshing. You'll have to find a few common Vietnamese/Thai staple ingredients like lemongrass and fish sauce, but once you know where to get your hands on them, they'll serve you time and time again. The fresh lemongrass (which can sometimes be found frozen) provides a distinctive gingery, citrus zip, while the fish sauce, or nuoc mam, provides a smoky, salty flavor that really can't be replicated. The flavors meld deliciously when combined with steak and cucumber in these tasty cups. Your family and friends will be particularly impressed with the presentation! Just keep in mind that the steak will need to marinate for at least 4 hours, or overnight if you are that organized.

MAKES 16 TO 18 CUPS

STEPS

❶ Combine the lemongrass, garlic, chili pepper, sugar, nuoc mam, vegetable oil, soy sauce, sesame oil, basil, and all mint except the garnish in a blender or food processor and pulse until mostly smooth. Some lumps will remain due to the lemongrass, which is perfectly normal.

❷ With a sharp knife, cut the steak into strips as thin as possible—think ¼ inch or less. (We'll be rough chopping the steak again once cooked, so don't fret if you can't slice it very thin.)

❸ Place the steak in a medium-size bowl and cover with all the marinade from step 1. Toss to coat the steak well. Cover with cling film and marinate for at least 4 hours, but no longer than 24, in the refrigerator.

❹ Remove the steak from the refrigerator and allow it to come to room temperature before cooking.

(recipe continues)

5 In a large sauté pan over medium-high heat, sauté the meat slices for approximately 5 minutes, until fully cooked, turning frequently as if you were stir-frying. Take off the heat and allow the meat to cool slightly.

6 Transfer the meat to a cutting board and dice into very small pieces with a sharp knife. Set aside.

7 Prepare the cucumber cups by peeling the cucumber and slicing into 1½-inch pieces (see photo).

8 With either a small melon baller or a small spoon, scoop out any seeds and create a small cavity in each cucumber piece, being careful not to accidentally break a hole in the bottom of the cup (see photo). Discard the seeds and extra flesh.

9 Fill the cucumber cups with the steak, pushing down slightly to pack in as much as possible (see photo).

10 Place on a serving platter, garnish with the reserved mint, and serve.

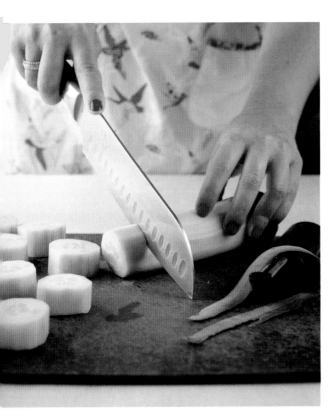

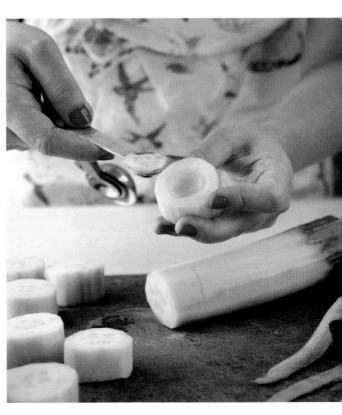

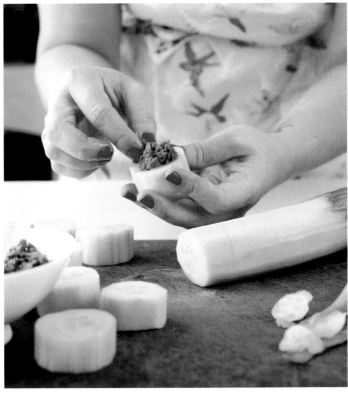

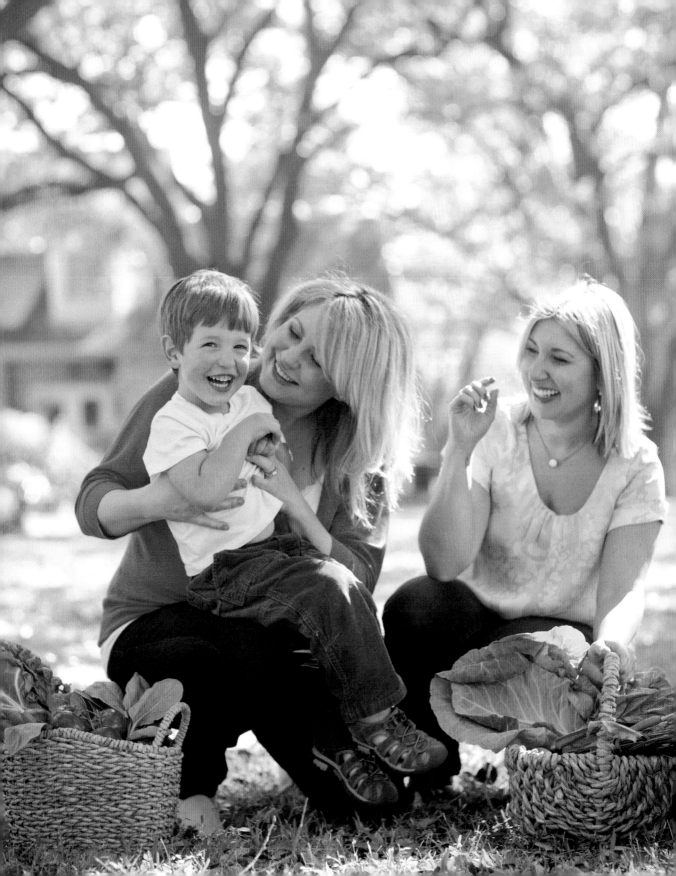

salads

At first thought, it doesn't seem to make much sense for us to feature a chapter of salads in a gluten-free cookbook, since salads are, most usually, naturally gluten-free. However, when at dinner parties or out at restaurants, we frequently have to choose a salad for our meal, as it's often the safest gluten-free bet. We have really acquired a strong affinity for salads of all kinds, and we thought it important to share some with you.

With so many varieties of lettuce, so many kinds of tomatoes, so many possible salad accoutrements, it was very difficult for us to narrow down the options to be included in this chapter. As you'll see, we tried to include some variations of the standard lettuce/tomato/something else version. We also attempted to stretch the conventional "salad" stereotype outside of the typical salad bowl by offering salads with noodles, beans, and different proteins. Some of these options are meals in and of themselves and offer a fantastic combination of healthy fats, lean proteins, and fiber-rich veggies. Others are better suited to serve at potlucks or parties in quantity. Whatever you are craving in terms of salad, there should certainly be something here to whet your appetite.

tuna salad niçoise
with **herb vinaigrette**

While Jilly was visiting Bruges, Belgium, she ate a version of this salad at least once a day. It seemed a healthy way to counterbalance all the delicious Belgian chocolate she had indulged in. Bruges is one of the most beautiful places on Earth, and anytime she makes this salad it brings back all the fond memories of her time spent there. We should warn you that no matter how delicious this recipe is, it does take a bit of prep time. If you want to save time, you can always cook the beans, potatoes, and eggs in advance. These ingredients make the dish hearty enough to serve as a filling meal. (Husbands agree, we can assure you.) Traditionally, anchovy fillets would also be included. Do feel free to use the anchovies if you like; just add 12 anchovy fillets. This salad is so easy on the eyes you'll almost not want to eat the beautiful masterpiece you've made. To step things up even more, try adding shredded pieces of freshly grilled tuna steaks instead of the canned variety.

SERVES 4

INGREDIENTS

salad

4 large eggs

1 pound green beans, ends trimmed

1 pound baby new potatoes, cut into bite-size chunks

¾ cup black olives, pitted and halved

½ cup cherry tomatoes, halved

½ cup yellow teardrop tomatoes, halved

½ small red onion, thinly sliced

7 ounces (usually one can) good-quality tuna, drained

1 teaspoon dried basil

Salt and black pepper to taste

Herb Vinaigrette (recipe follows)

herb vinaigrette

¼ cup white wine vinegar

1½ teaspoons herbs (mix of dried herbs such as thyme, marjoram, basil, garlic, and tarragon; use any combination you like)

Pinch of granulated sugar

Salt and black pepper to taste

2 teaspoons Dijon mustard

¾ cup extra virgin olive oil

STEPS

salad

❶ In a small saucepan of salted boiling water, boil the eggs for 8 to 10 minutes. Drain and set aside to cool.

❷ In a medium-size saucepan of salted boiling water, blanch the green beans until al dente, about 4 to 6 minutes, depending on size. Be careful to not overcook the beans; you want them still to have a bite.

❸ While the beans are cooking, fill a medium-size bowl with water and ice cubes. Remove the beans from the boiling water and shock them in the ice bath to stop them from cooking any further.

❹ Drain the beans and lay on a paper towel–lined plate to absorb excess liquid. Let cool.

❺ In another saucepan of salted boiling water, boil the potato chunks until fork tender, about 10 to 12 minutes, depending on size.

6 Drain the potatoes once cooked and allow them to cool.

7 Meanwhile, peel the eggs and cut into quarters.

8 Once the beans and potatoes are fully cooled, begin to assemble the salad: on a large plate or serving platter arrange the potatoes as the bottom layer.

9 Layer the green beans over the potatoes.

10 Scatter the olives, tomatoes, and red onions over the top.

11 Arrange the quartered egg slices around the edge of the plate.

12 Using your hands, flake the tuna over the salad.

13 Sprinkle the dried basil and a bit of salt and pepper over all.

14 Drizzle the Herb Vinaigrette on top of the salad to your personal preference of moistness and serve immediately.

herb vinaigrette

1 In a medium-size bowl, whisk together the vinegar, herbs, sugar, salt, and pepper.

2 Whisk in the Dijon mustard and gradually start to drizzle in the oil in a slow and steady stream, whisking continuously.

3 Once the dressing is emulsified and slightly thickened, taste and re-season if desired.

waldorf-style salad

INGREDIENTS

1 cup low-fat Greek-style yogurt

½ cup crumbled blue cheese, such as Cabrales

¼ cup lemon juice

¼ cup mayonnaise

2 tablespoons chopped parsley

2 teaspoons honey

2 teaspoons grated lemon zest

2 teaspoons salt

1 teaspoon freshly ground black pepper

5 large Honey Crisp apples

5 ribs celery from the heart, thinly sliced on the bias, leaves reserved for garnish

1 cup whole almonds, toasted and chopped

½ cup dried sour cherries, chopped

1 head Bibb lettuce, washed and dried, leaves separated

Recipe courtesy Emeril Lagasse, copyright MSLO, Inc., all rights reserved.

This is not your normal run-of-the-mill Waldorf-style salad, but then again, nothing our dad ever makes is run of the mill. Yes, the apples and celery you are accustomed to are here. But so are delicious crumbled blue cheese, crunchy almonds, tangy Greek yogurt, and sour cherries. This easy-to-make salad will impress any salad lover you know, so give it a try!

SERVES 8

STEPS

❶ In a small bowl combine the yogurt, blue cheese, lemon juice, mayonnaise, parsley, honey, lemon zest, salt, and pepper.

❷ Halve, core, and cut the apples into ¾-inch chunks, leaving the skin intact.

❸ Combine the apples, celery, almonds, and sour cherries in a bowl. Toss with the yogurt dressing.

❹ Arrange 8 lettuce leaves on salad plates; place the salad in the lettuce leaf, garnish with celery leaves, and serve immediately.

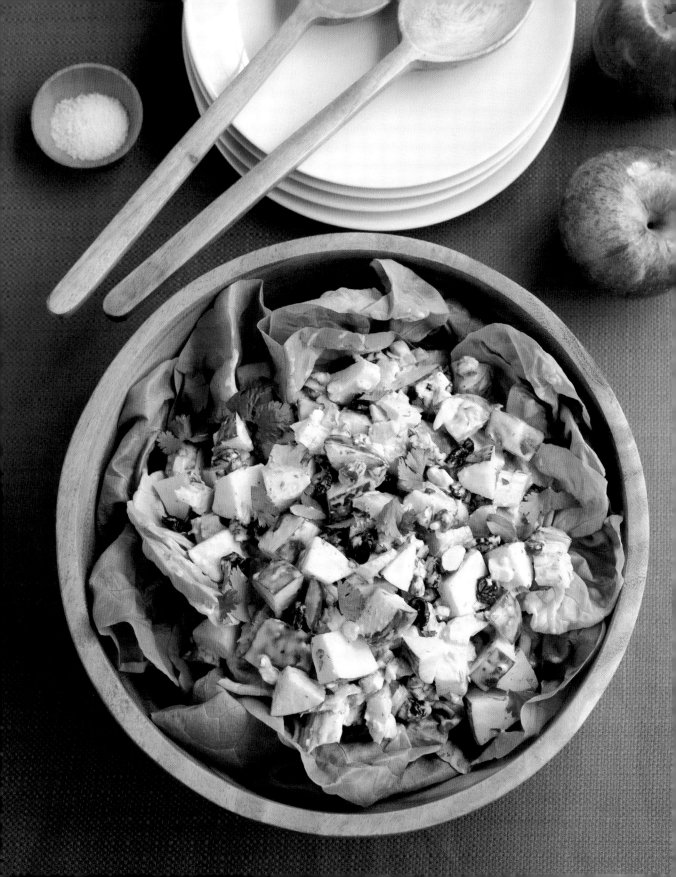

dill potato salad

INGREDIENTS

2 pounds baby new potatoes, cut into bite-size chunks

½ teaspoon Emeril's Original Essence Seasoning or Cajun seasoning of your choice

Pinch of celery salt

Salt and black pepper to taste

2 medium eggs, hard-boiled, peeled, and then chopped

½ large English cucumber or 1 medium-size regular cucumber, peeled, seeded, and chopped

½ small red onion, finely chopped

3 tablespoons finely chopped fresh dill

1 tablespoon finely chopped fresh mint

¼ cup Dijon mustard

3 tablespoons mayonnaise

This is a wonderful accompaniment to so many dishes: a nice juicy steak, a piece of grilled salmon, or roasted chicken. It will pair well with anything your heart desires. We must say fresh dill makes all the difference. You can substitute dried dill in a pinch; just be sure to remember the general rule for dried versus fresh herbs, that whatever you would use in tablespoons for fresh herbs, use only a teaspoon amount for dried herbs. This is because the dried herbs are more concentrated in potency. For a nice twist and a snappier taste, you could try substituting fresh tarragon for the mint. We prefer to use the Dijon mustard that contains seeds, but feel free to use whatever you have available. You can't go wrong either way.

SERVES 4

STEPS

1 In a medium-size saucepan of boiling salted water, cook the potato chunks until fork tender. Drain immediately and set aside to cool in a large bowl.

2 When the potatoes have cooled, season with the Essence Seasoning, celery salt, and a bit of salt and pepper.

3 Add the chopped eggs, cucumber, red onion, herbs, Dijon mustard, and mayonnaise and stir together gently until mixed well.

4 Taste and re-season as desired. If the salad is too dry for your liking, you can add a bit more mayonnaise.

5 Cover with cling film and chill in the refrigerator until ready to serve.

spring mix salad *with* pecans, apples, *and* buttermilk dressing

INGREDIENTS

salad

4 to 5 cups spring mix greens

1 medium-size apple, cored and thinly sliced

½ cup pecans, chopped

Buttermilk Dressing (recipe follows)

buttermilk dressing

¼ cup cider vinegar

¼ cup sour cream

¼ cup buttermilk

4 teaspoons finely minced green onion

1 tablespoon granulated sugar

1 teaspoon minced garlic

Salt and black pepper to taste

½ cup extra virgin olive oil

This is such an easy and delicious salad to prepare. The sweetness of the apples, the crunch of the pecans, and the creaminess of the dressing really complement the tartness of the lettuces. Although a pre-combined, prepackaged spring mix works well in this salad, you can use any tart salad green like radicchio or arugula just as effectively. We recommend using a sweet apple like a Fuji or Gala to balance the other flavors in this salad. A word of warning to all you heavy-handed dressing lovers: try not to use too much dressing or you'll overpower even the tartness of these greens!

SERVES 4 TO 6

STEPS

salad

❶ In a large salad bowl, combine the greens, apple, and pecans.

❷ Add the Buttermilk Dressing to the salad greens, but only enough to just coat the leaves. Toss so that all ingredients are distributed, and serve.

buttermilk dressing

❶ In a small bowl, whisk together the vinegar, sour cream, buttermilk, green onion, sugar, garlic, salt, and pepper until blended and creamy.

❷ Whisking constantly, slowly pour in the olive oil until the mixture emulsifies or thickens. It is important to add the oil in a slow, steady stream or else the whole dressing can "break" and it won't end up with the proper consistency.

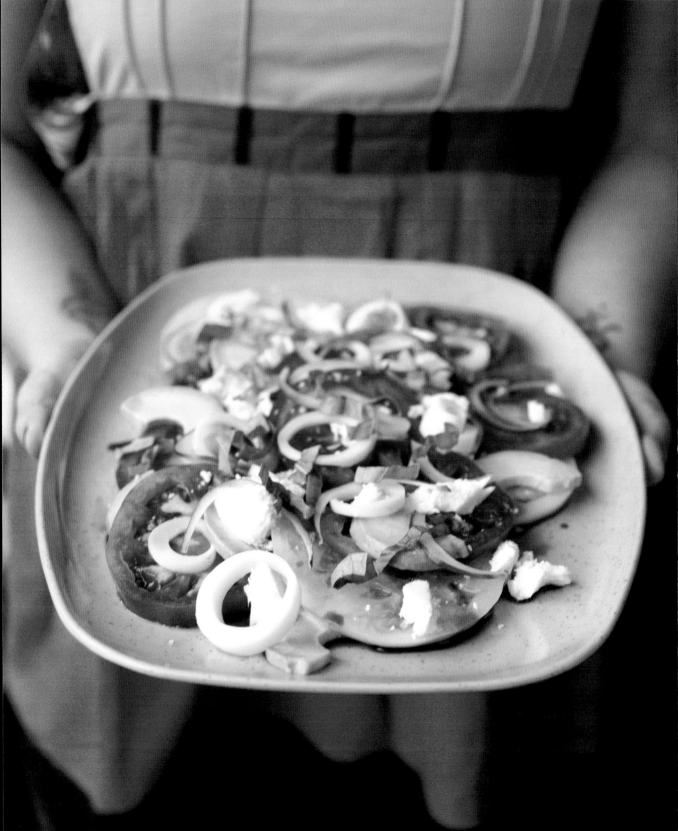

tomato layer salad

INGREDIENTS

2 large heirloom tomatoes, sliced

1 avocado, peeled, pitted, and sliced

6 ounces fresh mozzarella, sliced, about ¾ cup

½ small red onion, halved and thinly sliced

3 hearts of palm, sliced

½ teaspoon dried oregano or 1 to 1½ teaspoons finely chopped fresh oregano

Salt and black pepper to taste

1½ tablespoons finely chopped fresh basil

1½ tablespoons extra virgin olive oil

2 teaspoons balsamic vinegar

Recently, we discovered the wonderfully flavorful taste of heirloom tomatoes. There are hundreds of varieties of heirlooms out there, so you can use whatever kind you fancy most. Jessie developed this recipe because she needed to use up all the tomatoes in her garden! It's a wonderfully refreshing salad to serve chilled during those hot summer evenings. The order of the layers doesn't much matter as long as the tomatoes are on the bottom. Have some fun experimenting with different ordering or presentations for this easy yet tasty salad. You can also include some shrimp or tuna in the mix to add yet another dimension.

SERVES 4

STEPS

❶ On a large platter, arrange the sliced tomatoes to cover the bottom of the plate.

❷ On top of the tomatoes, make even layers of the slices of avocado, mozzarella cheese, onion, and hearts of palm.

❸ Season the entire dish with oregano, salt, and pepper.

❹ Sprinkle the chopped basil evenly over the entire dish. Lastly, drizzle the olive oil and balsamic vinegar over the whole plate and serve.

jessie's favorite greek salad

INGREDIENTS

¼ cup olive oil

3 tablespoons red wine vinegar

½ teaspoon dried oregano

½ teaspoon salt

¼ teaspoon black pepper

2 heads romaine lettuce, washed and dried

2 large fresh, ripe tomatoes, chopped (about 4 cups)

½ medium-size cucumber, peeled and sliced

½ medium-size green bell pepper, cored, seeded, and diced

1 medium-size red onion, thinly sliced (about 1½ cups)

1 cup Kalamata olives

1 cup crumbled feta cheese

There is a pizzeria in New Orleans that Jessie used to love to visit before she was diagnosed as gluten intolerant. Their pizza and house Greek salad are known for being consistently delicious. Even though she doesn't eat the pizza anymore, Jessie still visits *just* for the salad! Usually we don't like soggy salad greens, but this one tastes even better if you let the lettuce soak in the other ingredients for a while. We prefer to take the extra time to remove the ribs from the lettuce, but it is by no means required. Also, red wine vinegar has a strong flavor, so feel free to adjust the amount you use to suit your taste.

SERVES 6 TO 8

STEPS

❶ In a small bowl, whisk the olive oil, vinegar, oregano, salt, and black pepper until well blended.

❷ Tear the lettuce into bite-size pieces and place in a large salad bowl along with the tomatoes, cucumber, bell pepper, onion, and olives.

❸ Toss the salad with the dressing.

❹ Add the feta immediately before serving.

green bean *and* anchovy salad

INGREDIENTS

Salt

1 pound French green beans, topped and tailed

1½ tablespoons olive oil

1 tablespoon unsalted butter

1 shallot or small onion, thinly sliced

1 clove garlic, crushed

12 anchovy fillets, drained and roughly chopped

5 cremini, or baby bella, mushrooms, brushed clean and roughly sliced

Salt and black pepper to taste

2 tablespoons crème fraîche or full-fat sour cream

1 heaping tablespoon good-quality French whole-grain mustard

This is another dish we picked up in our travels, a taste of summer in the South of France that makes a delicious accompaniment to any gluten-free meal. This dish is probably best served alongside a nice juicy steak. For a lighter option, it also pairs well with your favorite white-fleshed fish. The saltiness of the anchovies is a great counterbalance to the fragrant green beans and mushrooms, while the tartness of the mustard helps to cut any fishiness. This savory salad is packed with salty, tangy flavors. It's simple and rustic, yet still elegant. We guarantee it will please your palate whether you are an anchovy lover or not. Serve warm or cold—the option is yours. Feel free to omit the mushrooms if desired.

SERVES 4

STEPS

❶ Fill a medium-size saucepan three-quarters full of salted water and bring to a rolling boil.

❷ Blanch the green beans in the boiling water until slightly tender, about 3 to 4 minutes. Be careful to not overcook the beans. You want them to be al dente.

❸ While the beans are cooking, fill a medium-size bowl with cold water and ice cubes.

❹ Drain the beans and shock them in the ice-water bath to stop them from cooking any further.

❺ After 2 minutes drain the beans again and lay on paper towels to absorb excess moisture.

❻ Add the oil and butter to the same pan and set over medium heat. When the butter begins to

melt, add the shallot and garlic and cook for 3 minutes.

❼ Add the anchovies, mushrooms, and a bit of salt and pepper and stir well. Cook another 3 minutes, until the mushrooms start to soften.

❽ Add the green beans, crème fraîche, mustard, and a bit more pepper, if desired. Stir well.

❾ Turn the heat down to low and cook 1 to 2 minutes longer, stirring well to mix all the ingredients.

❿ Remove from the heat and transfer the bean mixture to a serving bowl or dish. Serve immediately, if desired, or let the salad cool to room temperature.

grilled halloumi
and watermelon salad

INGREDIENTS

½ small red onion, thinly sliced

Juice of 1 lime

4 cups arugula, or rocket, salad leaves (about 2½ ounces)

8 ounces halloumi cheese, cut into ¼-inch slices

2 cups seedless watermelon, cut into bite-size chunks

⅓ cup fresh mint leaves, finely chopped

1 tablespoon extra virgin olive oil

This dish was created in homage to Jilly's best friend in London, Ashley, who describes herself as a halloumi-aholic. She adores this dish so much that Jilly had to promise she would dedicate the recipe to her. So, here you go, my love! Halloumi is a delicious Cypriot cheese usually made from goat or sheep's milk. Also known as the squeaky cheese, halloumi is quite salty in flavor and has a very high melting point, making it perfect for barbecuing, grilling, or frying. Because of this unique quality, there isn't really a substitute for halloumi, although you could use feta cheese, ungrilled, for another take. It will still make for a great salad, though perhaps not as standout as the original. If you can, try this summertime treat at your next barbecue and discover the deliciousness of halloumi for yourself. Ashley claims a summer barbecue just isn't the same without it!

SERVES 2 TO 4

STEPS

❶ In a small bowl combine the red onion and lime juice and let stand for 15 minutes. This lets the acid in the citrus juice sweeten the onion naturally.

❷ On a large plate or serving platter, arrange the arugula leaves evenly to create a base for the dish.

❸ Heat either a griddle or a sauté pan over medium heat. Once the griddle or pan is hot, grill or fry the cheese until golden in color, about 4 to 5 minutes on each side. Turn off the heat and set aside.

❹ Drain any liquid from the red onions

❺ Arrange the watermelon, red onions, and grilled halloumi on top of the greens.

❻ Sprinkle the salad with the mint. Drizzle the olive oil over all to finish. Serve immediately.

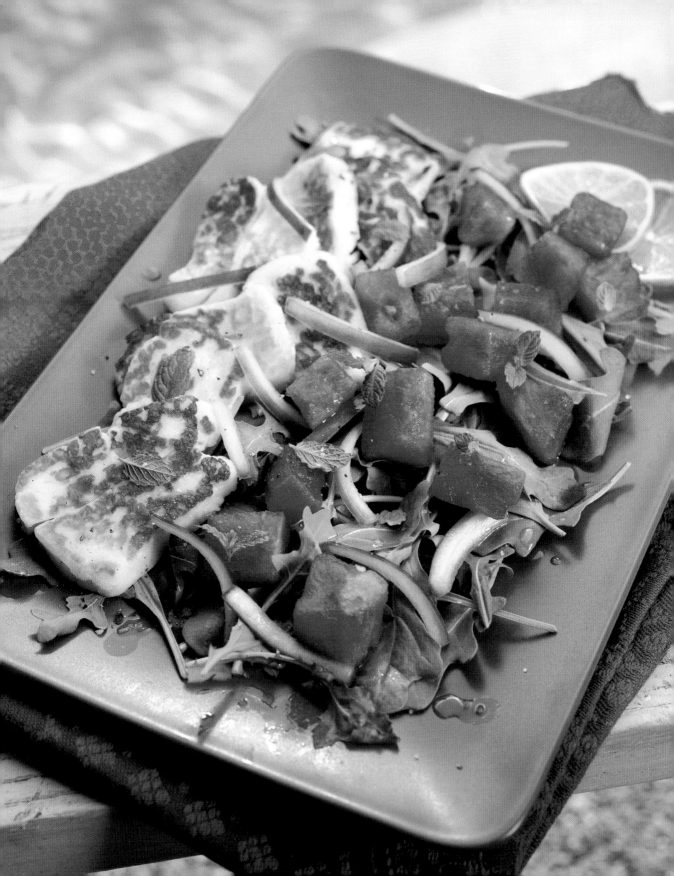

pear *and* fennel salad *with* goat cheese *and* candied walnuts

INGREDIENTS

salad

Walnut Dressing (recipe follows)

3 small pears, any variety, cored and cut into bite-size pieces

1 lemon, halved

1 tablespoon unsalted butter

½ cup walnut halves

1 tablespoon (packed) light brown sugar

1 head endive or chicory lettuce, washed and patted dry

1 large or 2 medium bulbs fresh fennel, trimmed of tough outer layer, quartered lengthwise, and thinly sliced (about 2 cups)

½ small red onion, thinly sliced

Salt and black pepper to taste

4 ounces good-quality goat cheese (chèvre)

1 teaspoon fresh thyme leaves, roughly chopped

walnut dressing

2 tablespoons white or red wine vinegar

½ teaspoon finely grated orange zest

Pinch of salt and black pepper to taste

Pinch of granulated sugar

3 tablespoons walnut oil or any light salad oil

The delicate flavors of the pear and the fennel, combined with the creamy goat cheese and sweet, crunchy candied walnuts, make for an elegant and refined salad, sure to please any palate. Yet you'll be amazed at how easy it is to prepare. Fennel is one of our favorite salad additions, with its strong aniseed/licorice flavor. It adds such an interesting depth to this dish. Just make sure to peel off and discard any discolored outer part of the bulb and the base or stem, which can be bitter in taste. We like to serve this as a starter or appetizer at dinner parties, which always seems to impress. Try it for yourselves.

SERVES 4

STEPS

salad

❶ First prepare the Walnut Dressing and set aside.

❷ In a medium-size nonstick skillet over medium heat, cook the sliced pears for 2 minutes to slightly soften.

❸ Remove from the heat and place the pears in a large bowl. Drizzle with juice from half the lemon to prevent browning, toss gently to coat, and set aside.

❹ In the same skillet, melt the butter over medium-low heat. Add the walnuts and brown sugar and stir well to coat. Cook, stirring occasionally, until the nuts are crisp, about 4 to 5 minutes. Remove from the heat and set aside.

❺ Core the endive or chicory by taking a paring knife and, in a circular movement, carefully cutting around the bottom core. It should twist out. Peel the leaves off the core and add to the bowl.

❻ Add the fennel and red onion to the bowl and drizzle the juice from the remaining lemon half over all. Mix together well and season with salt and pepper.

❼ Add the toasted walnuts, goat cheese, and thyme to the bowl, drizzle with the dressing, and toss again until well mixed.

❽ Distribute the salad evenly among 4 individual plates. Serve immediately.

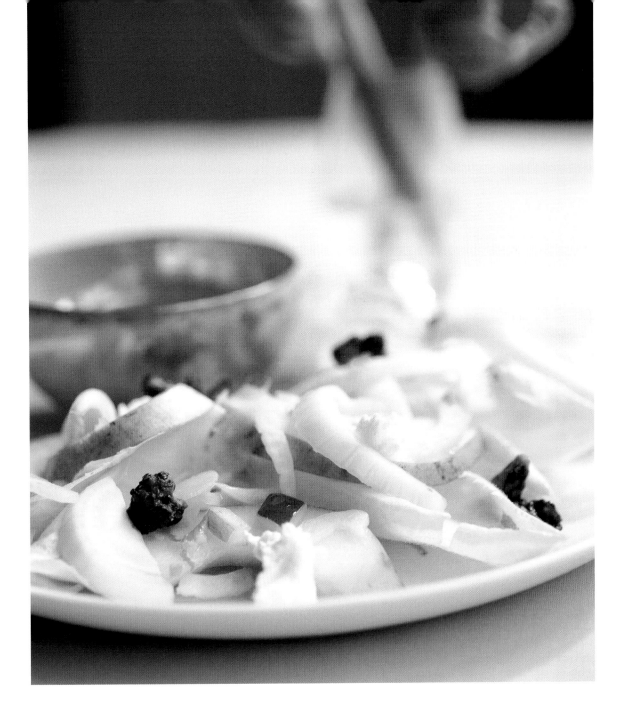

walnut dressing

❶ In a medium-size bowl, whisk together all of the dressing ingredients except the oil.

❷ Gradually drizzle in the oil in a slow and steady stream, whisking continuously until it starts to thicken and emulsify.

❸ Taste and re-season, if desired. Set aside until ready to use.

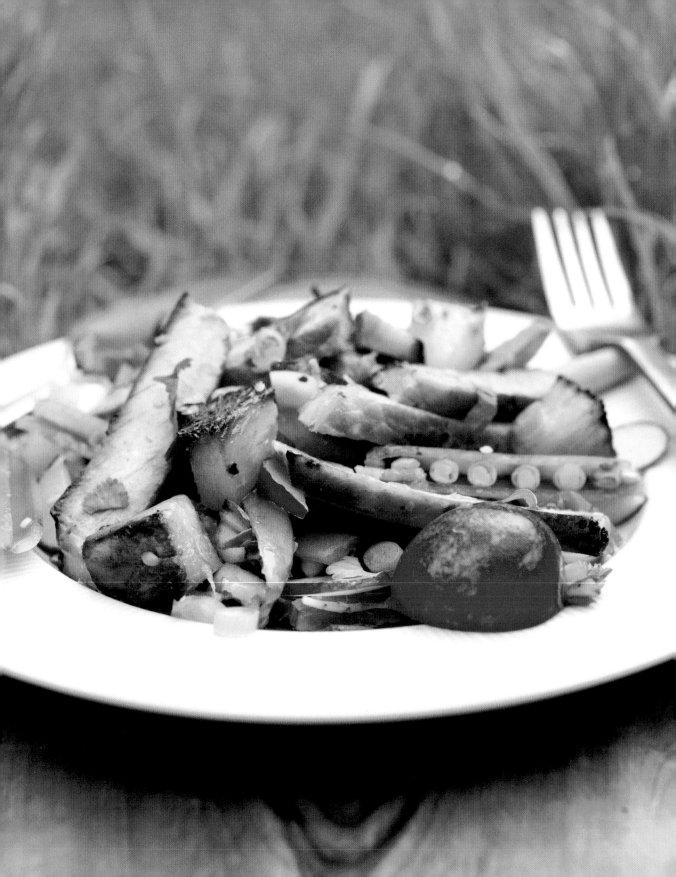

garlic pork *with* oriental salad

INGREDIENTS

2 tablespoons toasted sesame oil, plus additional if needed

1 tablespoon vegetable oil

2 lean pork chops, boneless variety preferred

1 can (8 ounces) pineapple chunks, drained

1 clove garlic, crushed

Pinch of crushed red pepper flakes

Salt and black pepper to taste

6 small radishes, thinly sliced

1 cup sugar snap peas, sliced into long, thin strips (about 4 ounces)

1 small head green bok choy, leaves finely chopped and stems finely shredded

¼ cup chopped fresh cilantro

Juice and finely grated zest of one large lemon

2 teaspoons gluten-free soy sauce or tamari

2 teaspoons honey

4 small green onions, thinly sliced on the diagonal

We seem to have loads of scrumptious recipes in the book that are capable of feeding a small army. But what about the nights when it's just the two of you and neither of you really wants leftovers? For nights like these, here is the perfect meal for two. This dish just dances on your palate with the tang, the sweet, the spice. Not only is it packed full of your recommended five-a-day fruit and vegetable servings, but it is quite filling as well. If you don't like pineapple, substitute any variety of orange you enjoy, or feel free to barbecue the pork without it. Or add thinly sliced matchsticks of apple to the salad for a different twist. If you want a more filling take on this dish, serve some cooked rice noodles or steamed rice alongside.

SERVES 2

STEPS

❶ In a medium-size sauté pan, heat 1 tablespoon of the sesame oil and the vegetable oil over medium-high heat.

❷ Add the pork chops, pineapple chunks, garlic, crushed red pepper flakes, and salt and black pepper. Cook for 6 to 7 minutes, turning the chops over once to make sure they are fully cooked through. If your pork is quite thick, it might take a few minutes longer to cook. If so, and if necessary, you can add more sesame oil to keep the ingredients from burning in the pan.

❸ Turn off the heat and cover the pan to keep warm.

❹ In a medium-size bowl, combine the radishes, sugar snap peas, bok choy, and cilantro.

❺ In a small bowl, whisk together the remaining 1 tablespoon sesame oil, lemon juice and zest, gluten-free soy sauce or tamari, and honey to make a dressing.

❻ Drizzle the dressing over the vegetables in the bowl, add salt and black pepper to taste, if desired, and toss well.

❼ While the pork is still warm, remove the chops from the pan to a cutting board and cut into thick slices, about 6 per chop, depending on size. Add to the bowl of salad, along with the pineapple chunks and juices from the pan.

❽ Add the green onions to the salad and toss all together well. Serve immediately.

satay chicken salad
with **rice noodles**

INGREDIENTS

salad

2 large boneless, skinless chicken breasts

1 can (14 ounces) coconut milk

Spicy Satay Sauce (recipe follows)

1 large carrot, peeled, halved, and cut into thin matchsticks

½ cup diagonally halved snow peas (about 2 ounces)

1 package (8 ounces) rice noodles

½ English cucumber, peeled, seeded, halved lengthwise, and cut into matchsticks

1 red bell pepper, cored, seeded, and cut into long, thin strips

½ cup bean sprouts, washed and patted dry

4 sprigs fresh cilantro, leaves only, roughly chopped

3 sprigs fresh mint, leaves only, finely chopped

1 sprig fresh Thai basil, leaves only, roughly chopped

2 green onions, sliced diagonally

Salt and black pepper (optional)

This is our take on those gorgeous rice-paper rolls you can get in your favorite Thai or Vietnamese restaurant. They are healthy and delicious, fresh and cooling. After more attempts than we care to admit trying to master the art of rolling spring rolls ourselves, we admitted defeat. So instead, what we've done is turn all the good stuff inside the rolls out! This dish is exploding with vibrant flavors, from the spicy, nutty satay sauce to the cooling mint, cucumber, and delicate coconut-steamed chicken.

SERVES 4 TO 6

STEPS

salad

❶ Place the chicken in a medium-size saucepan and cover with the coconut milk. If the chicken isn't covered fully, add water to the pan until it is.

❷ Bring the liquid to a simmer over medium heat. Reduce the heat to medium-low, cover the pan with a lid, and poach the chicken until fully cooked through about 30 to 40 minutes, depending on size.

❸ While the chicken is cooking, prepare the Spicy Satay Sauce and refrigerate until ready to use.

❹ Once the chicken is fully cooked, turn off the heat, uncover, and allow the chicken to cool in the coconut poaching liquid.

❺ While the chicken is cooling, bring salted water to a rolling boil in a small saucepan and prepare a bowl of ice water.

❻ Blanch the carrots and snow peas for 1 minute in the boiling water. Immediately drain and place them in the ice-water bath for 2 minutes to shock them. Drain the vegetables again and lay them on a paper towel–lined plate to dry. Set aside to cool.

(recipe continues)

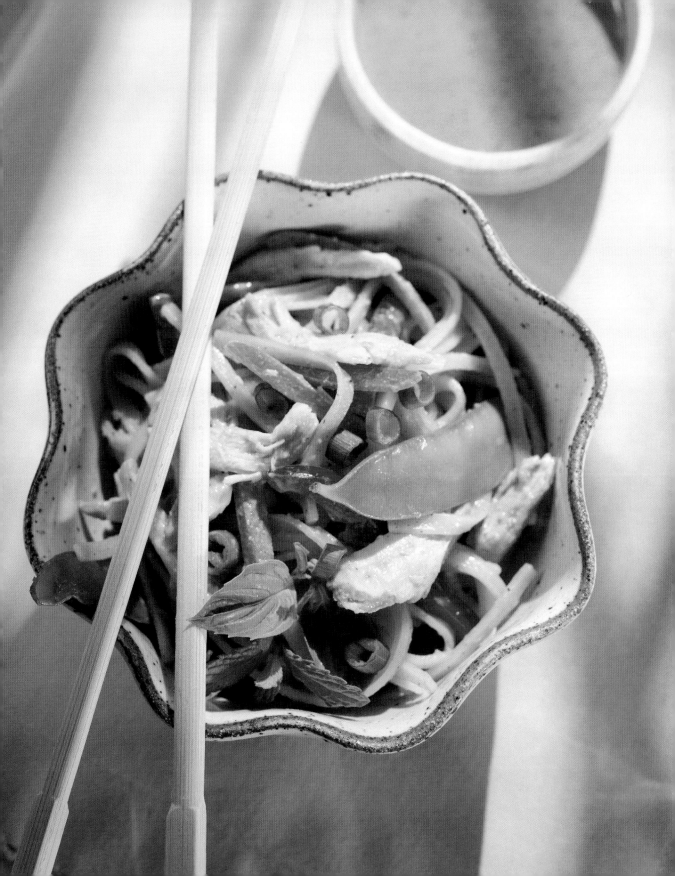

INGREDIENTS (CONT.)

spicy satay sauce

¼ cup plus 2 tablespoons coconut milk or cream

½ small red onion, chopped

1 clove garlic, crushed

¼ cup smooth peanut butter, any you like

2 teaspoons (packed) light brown sugar

2 teaspoons gluten-free soy sauce or tamari

½ teaspoon chili powder

Drizzle of honey (roughly 1 tablespoon)

Pinch of salt and black pepper

STEPS (CONT.)

7 Prepare enough rice noodles for 4 to 6 appetizer portions as directed on the package. Set aside.

8 Once fully cooled, shred the chicken into small pieces, using your hands. Set aside while you start to assemble the salad.

9 On either 4 large individual plates or a large serving platter, make a layer of the warm rice noodles. With a knife, cut them roughly into smaller pieces. This will make them easier to manage when eating.

10 Spoon half the Spicy Satay Sauce over the noodles.

11 Layer the blanched carrots, snow peas, cucumber, red bell pepper, and bean sprouts over the noodles.

12 Layer the shredded chicken over the vegetables.

13 Scatter the chopped fresh herbs and green onions over all. Season with salt and pepper, if desired.

14 Spoon the remaining half of the satay sauce over the chicken and vegetables, toss all gently to mix, and serve.

spicy satay sauce

1 Combine all the ingredients for the sauce in a food processor or blender and puree until smooth.

2 Spoon the sauce into a small bowl, cover with cling film, and place in the refrigerator until needed.

wilted spinach salad
with bacon vinegar dressing

INGREDIENTS

8 slices bacon, diced

3 tablespoons apple cider vinegar

½ teaspoon granulated sugar

¼ teaspoon black pepper, plus more as desired

8 cups baby spinach (10 to 12 ounces), washed and patted dry

1 cup diced yellow onion

1½ teaspoons minced garlic

Salt to taste

Jessie first had a salad similar to this when she was in northern Italy. This version has a lot less bacon fat than the one she remembers, but it still has enough to lend its distinctive bacon-y flavor to the dressing—just enough to feel indulgent! Spinach wilts very quickly, so be sure to have everything prepped and ready before you begin tossing the salad. Also, some bacon has a high salt content, so be sure to sample the salad after tossing before adding any more salt.

SERVES 6

STEPS

❶ Fry the diced bacon in a medium-size skillet over medium-high heat until crispy, about 10 to 12 minutes.

❷ While the bacon is cooking, mix the vinegar, sugar, and pepper together in a small bowl and set aside. Place the spinach in a large bowl and set it aside as well.

❸ Once the bacon is crispy, remove from the skillet with a slotted spoon to a plate covered with paper towels. This will help soak up excess grease.

❹ Pour off and discard all but approximately 3 tablespoons of the bacon grease from the skillet.

❺ Replace the skillet on the stove. Sauté the onion and garlic over medium heat until the onion is soft, about 3 to 5 minutes.

❻ Stir in the vinegar mixture and remove the skillet from the heat.

❼ Pour the dressing over the spinach, add the bacon pieces, and re-season with salt and pepper to taste. Toss gently with tongs to mix and coat the spinach leaves. Serve immediately.

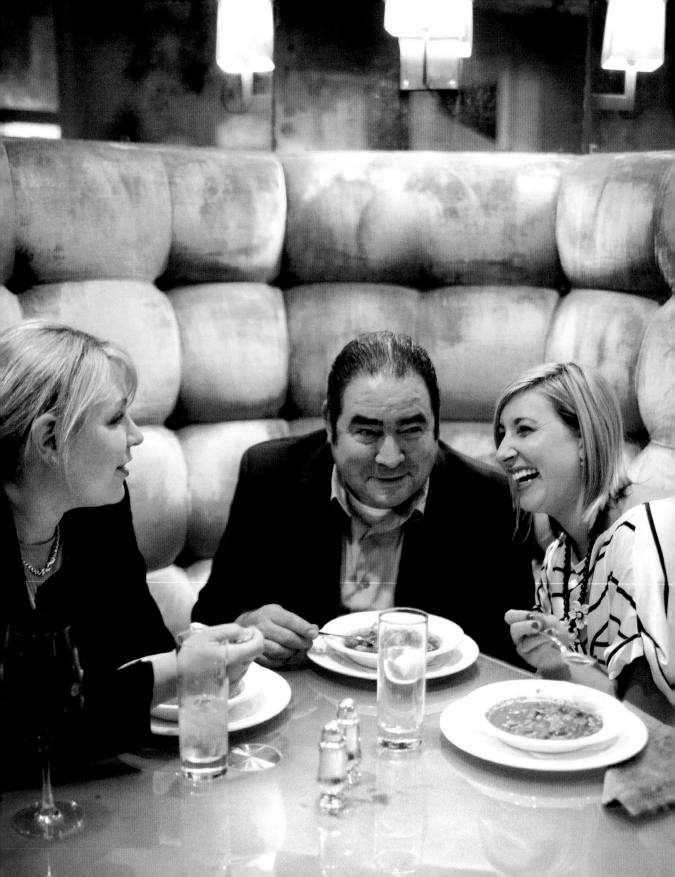

soups

There is nothing more comforting to us than a wonderfully warm and aromatic bowl of soup. We spent most of our young lives whiling away the frigid winters in southeastern Massachusetts, a place where a crock full of hot soup was most appreciated! Soups, more than any other type of dish, tend to elicit fond childhood memories for us, perhaps because the memory-triggering smells so effortlessly transport us back to our youth. Our great-grandmother, Grandma Cabral, used to make a delicious kale and chorizo soup that we still crave even after all these years. She'd unfailingly have some ready for us when we stopped in for a visit after sledding or ice skating. We never could quite crack her recipe for that soup; otherwise we would have shared it with you all here! Despite its absence, we did include a variety of tummy-pleasing memory-makers for you to try. Cozy up with your spouse, kids, or pets and enjoy!

aldie's tortilla soup

INGREDIENTS

3 tablespoons olive oil

1 green bell pepper, cored, seeded, and chopped

1 medium-size yellow onion, chopped

Salt

1 pound lean ground turkey

½ teaspoon ground cumin

½ teaspoon ground coriander

¼ teaspoon chili powder, plus more if desired

1 clove garlic, minced

Black pepper

1 can (15 ounces) black beans, undrained

1 can (10 ounces) diced tomatoes with green chilies

1 cup corn kernels, drained

6 cups vegetable or chicken stock

1 cup water

Chopped fresh cilantro leaves, for garnish

1 ripe Hass avocado, peeled, pitted, and cut into bite-size cubes, for garnish

Good-quality 100% corn tortilla chips or strips, for serving

Our stepmother, Aldie, is an incredible cook—you simply have to be to get respect in this family! This is Jilly's take on Aldie's famous tortilla soup, which is naturally gluten-free and one of our favorite things in her repertoire. Not only is it a superbly easy one-pot wonder, and one of the most filling fiestas you can find in any bowl, but it's also extremely healthy. Simple, nutritious, and delicious—a triple threat! Feel free to substitute lean ground beef for the turkey and get adventurous with the toppings. Jessie likes a nice dollop of sour cream on hers.

SERVES 8 TO 10

STEPS

1 In a large (8-quart) stockpot over medium heat, heat the olive oil.

2 Add the bell pepper and onion and sauté with a bit of salt for 5 minutes, until the vegetables are softened.

3 Add the turkey and cook, crumbling with a wooden spoon, until the meat loses its raw look and is beginning to brown, about 8 minutes.

4 Add the spices, garlic, and salt and black pepper to taste.

5 Add the black beans with their liquid, the diced tomatoes with chilies, and the corn.

6 Add the stock and water, stir well, and bring to a simmer over medium heat.

7 Reduce the heat to medium-low and cook, uncovered, for 20 minutes, making sure the soup never boils.

8 Turn off the heat. Taste and re-season as needed.

9 Serve in bowls and garnish each with a sprinkle of cilantro, some of the avocado, and a generous handful of tortilla chips on top.

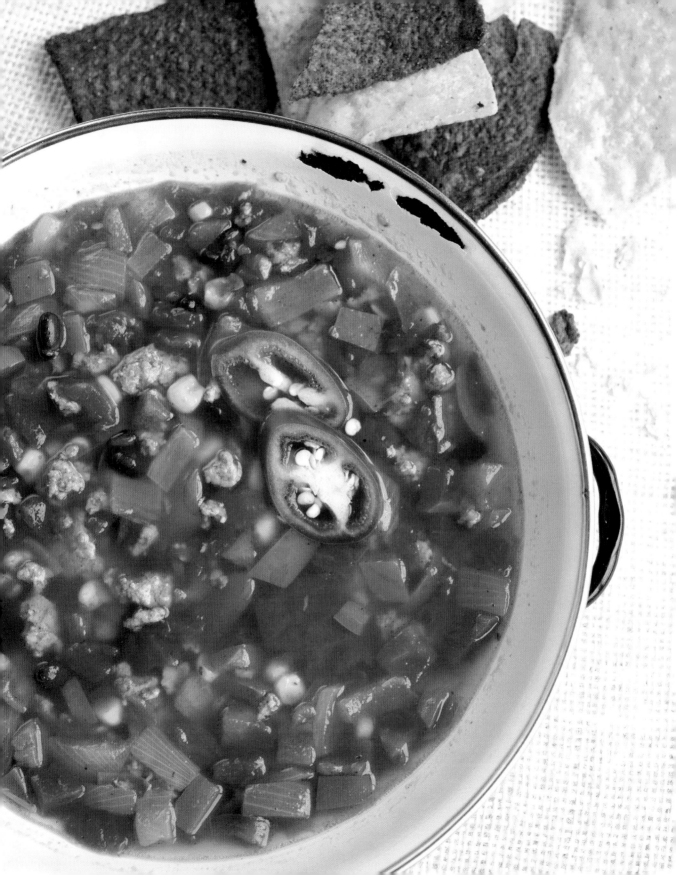

crab *and* corn bisque

INGREDIENTS

2 tablespoons olive oil

1 tablespoon lightly salted butter

1 cup diced yellow onion

1 red bell pepper, cored, seeded, and diced

1 cup finely chopped celery

2 cloves garlic, minced

½ teaspoon celery salt

1½ teaspoons Emeril's Original Essence Seasoning or Old Bay Seasoning

Salt and black pepper to taste

⅓ cup cornstarch

5 cups vegetable or seafood stock

2 large potatoes, peeled and cut into small bite-size chunks

1 can (11 ounces) corn kernels

2 bay leaves

2 cups half-and-half

Generous pinch of cayenne pepper

1 pound jumbo lump crabmeat, picked over for shells

Finely chopped fresh chives, for garnish

This truly decadent soup will be a real show stopper at your next dinner party or holiday gathering. Unlike in most creamy soups, cornstarch is used instead of a wheat-flour roux to thicken it. Try to buy the highest-quality crabmeat that is available to you; it makes a big difference. You can freeze any leftovers that you have, though we doubt you'll be able to hold back! Crab and Corn Bisque is easily our mother's most oft-requested dish whenever Jilly is home visiting. One taste of this sweet and sophisticated soup and you'll know why. We personally love to pair this with Against The Grain Gourmet's baguettes. Yum!

SERVES 10 TO 12

STEPS

1 In a large (8-quart) stockpot over medium heat, heat the oil and butter.

2 Add the onion, bell pepper, celery, and garlic to the pot and stir well.

3 Cook the vegetables until they are slightly softened, about 6 to 8 minutes.

4 Add the celery salt, Essence Seasoning, and a bit of salt and black pepper and stir well.

5 In a small bowl or measuring cup, dissolve the cornstarch in 1 cup of the stock, stirring well to make sure any lumps are dissolved.

6 Add this mixture to the pot along with the remaining stock and stir well.

7 Add the potatoes, corn, and bay leaves to the pot, stir, and bring to a gentle boil over medium-high heat. Boil gently for 10 minutes.

8 Turn the heat down to low and simmer.

9 Add the half-and-half and cayenne pepper, and stir. Simmer a further 15 minutes uncovered, stirring occasionally. The bisque should now start to thicken up.

10 Add the crabmeat and continue to cook on low until the potatoes are cooked through or the crabmeat is heated through, whichever comes later.

11 Taste and re-season if needed before serving in bowls, garnished with a sprinkling of chopped chives.

beef stew

INGREDIENTS

1½ pounds beef stew meat

¼ cup gluten-free all-purpose flour blend (we've used Arrowhead Mills Gluten Free All Purpose Baking Mix)

1 teaspoon black pepper, plus more to taste

½ teaspoon salt, plus more to taste

3 cups chopped onion (about 2 large onions)

1 tablespoon minced garlic

3 tablespoons olive oil

1 cup dry red wine

8 cups beef stock

2 cups chopped carrot (4 medium-size or 2 large carrots, peeled)

4 medium-size red potatoes, peeled and cut into bite-size chunks

3 bay leaves

¼ cup fresh thyme leaves or 1½ teaspoons dried thyme

When we were considering a beef stew recipe for this book, we quickly realized that almost everyone has his or her own favorite, whether regional or something their family has passed down. We included this one because it's *our* favorite—it tastes great even gluten-free, and the broth is oh-so-perfect for dipping gluten-free French baguettes or gluten-free crackers! The red wine in this recipe adds a terrific depth of flavor, but try to use one that's pretty dry, since that's the one that ends up tasting the best.

SERVES 4 TO 6

STEPS

❶ Place the stew meat in a medium-size bowl. Toss with the flour blend, 1 teaspoon pepper, and ½ teaspoon salt until most, if not all, of the flour adheres to the meat. Set aside for a few minutes.

❷ In a medium-size (6-quart) stockpot, sauté the onion and garlic in the olive oil over medium heat until the onion begins to soften, 3 to 5 minutes..

❸ Add the meat to the pot and stir until the pieces are coated with the oil.

❹ Stir in the red wine, making sure to loosen all of the pieces of meat or onion that might have been stuck on the bottom of the pot. The flour should begin to thicken the liquid after a few minutes of heating.

❺ Add the beef stock and all the remaining ingredients. Stirring occasionally, simmer uncovered on medium-low for 40 minutes, or until the vegetables are tender. Re-season the stew as desired and serve.

french onion soup
with gruyère-smothered crostini

INGREDIENTS

2 tablespoons olive oil

3 pounds red onions, thinly
  sliced (about 10 cups)

Salt

4 sprigs fresh thyme

2 sprigs fresh parsley

4 cups chicken stock

4 cups beef stock

½ cup dry red wine

1 bay leaf

1 tablespoon balsamic vinegar

Black pepper to taste

1 gluten-free baguette, cut
  into ½- to ¾-inch slices

8 ounces Gruyère cheese,
  grated (about 2 cups)

Finely sliced green onions, for
  garnish (optional)

French onion soup has always been one of Jessie's favorite soups, especially when served with several soup-soaked cheesy crostini. This particular recipe highlights the flavor of red onions, but any type of onion can be used if there's one that you prefer or already have on hand. If you are lucky enough to have access to premade gluten-free baguettes, like the ones made by Against The Grain Gourmet, they will make perfect crostini for this recipe. If not, gluten-free-pizza crust, like the one made by Arrowhead Mills, can be shaped into baguette form and used instead. Another trick we learned with this recipe involves the herbs. It's a lot easier to fish the parsley and thyme out of the soup if you tie the sprigs together with some butcher's twine!

SERVES 6

STEPS

❶ Heat the olive oil in a large (8-quart) nonstick stockpot over medium-high heat for 1 to 2 minutes just to get the oil warm.

❷ Add the onions and about ½ teaspoon salt. Stir so that the oil coats all the onions.

❸ Cook for 30 to 40 minutes over medium heat, stirring the onions often. The onions will become caramelized and brownish and begin to form a syrupy crust on the bottom of the pan.

❹ Meanwhile, with butcher's twine, gently tie the stems of the thyme and parsley together to form a mini herb bouquet. Set aside.

❺ Once the onions are fully caramelized, stir in the chicken stock, beef stock, red wine, thyme-and-parsley-bouquet, and bay leaf. Loosen the browned crust on the pan's bottom with a spoon and stir until those bits become incorporated into the liquid.

❻ Bring the soup to a simmer and cook another 20 to 30 minutes to meld all of the flavors.

❼ Preheat the oven to broil.

❽ Remove the soup from the heat. Stir in the balsamic vinegar and add salt and black pepper as desired. Remove the herbs, including the bay leaf.

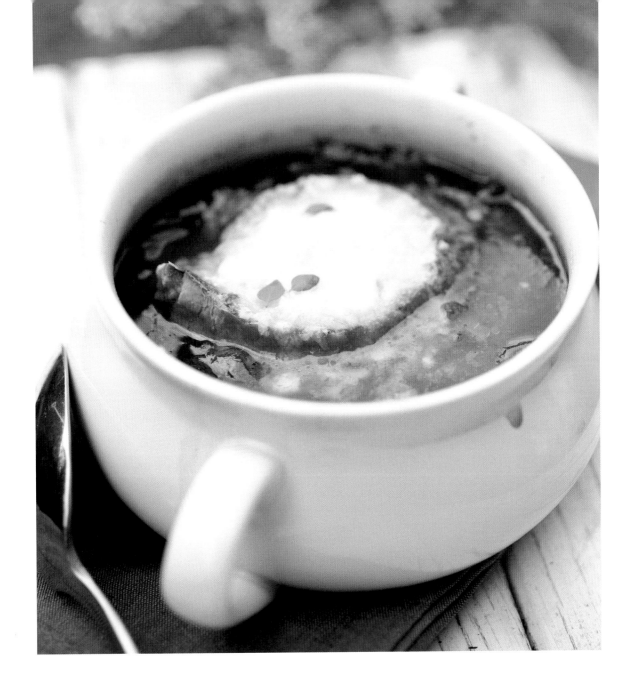

⑨ Ladle about 1 cup of soup into each of 6 ovenproof soup bowls and place on a baking tray.

⑩ Top the soup in each bowl with 1 to 2 slices of the baguette and sprinkle the bread with approximately ⅓ cup cheese.

⑪ Broil the soups until the cheese is bubbly and browned, about 3 to 5 minutes, depending on your oven.

⑫ Remove from the oven and garnish with green onions, if desired. Let cool for several minutes and serve.

chicken noodle soup

2 tablespoons olive oil

2 cups coarsely chopped onion (about 2 medium-size onions)

2 teaspoons minced garlic

1 cup thinly sliced carrot (2 medium-size or 1 large carrot, peeled)

½ cup diced celery

8 cups chicken stock

2 boneless, skinless chicken breasts, diced

2 cups frozen broccoli florets

2 teaspoons Emeril's Original Essence Seasoning or Cajun seasoning of your choice

2 bay leaves

½ teaspoon salt, plus more to taste

¼ teaspoon black pepper, plus more to taste

1 package (8 ounces) rice noodles

For years, whenever one of us was sick, we'd ask Dad to make us some "feel-good chicken soup." Whether it was the combination of spices or just plain coincidence, no one knows, but we always seemed to get better after just one or two big steaming bowls! Here's our gluten-free version, which is just as tasty as the original. Just remember to cook the noodles separately or else all of your soup stock will be sucked up into the noodles, leaving a big, gelatinous—although tasty—mess.

SERVES 6

STEPS

❶ Heat the oil in a large (8-quart) stockpot over medium heat. Add the onions and garlic and sauté for 5 to 7 minutes, or until the onions are tender.

❷ Add the carrot and celery and sauté a few minutes more, or until the celery begins to soften.

❸ Add all the remaining ingredients except for the rice noodles. Stirring occasionally, let the soup simmer for 30 minutes, or until the chicken is cooked through and all the veggies are soft.

❹ While the soup is simmering, prepare enough rice noodles for 4 servings as directed on the package.

❺ When the soup is ready, add the cooked rice noodles and simmer for another 5 minutes. Remove the bay leaves, re-season as desired, and serve.

kale *and* chickpea stew

INGREDIENTS

¼ cup ghee

1 medium-size yellow onion, chopped

2 cloves garlic, minced

2 teaspoons chopped fresh ginger

1 teaspoon freshly ground coriander seeds

1 teaspoon freshly ground cumin seeds

¾ teaspoon ground turmeric

¼ teaspoon cayenne pepper

¼ teaspoon whole yellow mustard seeds

1 pound kale, stems removed, leaves cut into bite-size pieces

2 large sweet potatoes, peeled and cut into 1-inch cubes

One can (19 ounces) chickpeas, drained

5 cups vegetable stock or canned low-sodium vegetable broth

1½ teaspoons kosher salt

1 cup canned unsweetened coconut milk

Cooked jasmine rice, for serving

2 tablespoons chopped cilantro, for garnish

¼ cup julienned red bell pepper, for garnish

Recipe courtesy Emeril Lagasse, copyright MSLO, Inc., all rights reserved.

This Indian-flavored stew is chock full of healthiness for you and your family! Kale, chickpeas, sweet potato, garlic, fresh ginger, *and* turmeric? Talk about superfoods…this is like a big bowl of superfood heaven! Some Indians say that the reason they don't get sick with colds or the flu is because of all the spices, ginger, and chilies they use in their cooking. We have to agree with that. Ghee is simply clarified butter frequently used in South Asian (Indian, Nepali, Bangladeshi, Pakistani) cuisine. You should be able to find it at your local grocery store in the Indian food section. If not, try your nearest specialty food store or Whole Foods Market. Try this winter warmer for yourselves and show that flu who is boss!

SERVES 4 TO 6

STEPS

1 In a large saucepan or Dutch oven, heat the ghee over medium heat. Add the onion and cook for 3 minutes, or until translucent.

2 Add the garlic and ginger and cook for another 2 minutes.

3 Add the coriander, cumin, turmeric, cayenne, and yellow mustard seeds and cook for 1 minute longer.

4 Add the kale, sweet potatoes, chickpeas, vegetable broth, and salt and increase the heat to medium high. As soon as the stew begins to simmer, reduce the heat to medium low and gently simmer for 35 minutes, or until the sweet potatoes are tender.

5 Stir in the coconut milk and cook for 15 minutes longer.

6 Serve with the jasmine rice and garnish with the chopped cilantro and red bell pepper.

note: *Turmeric is a rhizome that is used widely in Indian cooking. It is one of the main ingredients in curry, lending it a distinctive flavor. Turmeric has a slightly bitter flavor. It is used as a food coloring for cheese, butter, and mustard thanks to its bright yellow color. Turmeric is also considered a super antioxidant and is used in both Indian and Chinese herbal medicines.*

new orleans chicken
and sausage gumbo

Living in New Orleans, we have eaten a lot of gumbo in our day. But we have never taken it for granted, because we know firsthand that good gumbo requires lots of love and attention. Our father taught us at an early age how important a good roux is to making a successful gumbo! Traditionally, this would be a rich dark brown color, almost like chocolate. But gluten-free flour doesn't cook down exactly the same as wheat flour. Thus, your roux will stay light blond in color. It's perfectly normal and, we can guarantee, just as delicious. We also love the heat that a good spicy Cajun andouille sausage adds to this gumbo, though kielbasa would also work well. Just be sure to check your ingredients, as some sausages contain wheat flour to bind or bulk up the product. *Laissez les bons temps rouler*. Let the good times roll, y'all!

SERVES 6 TO 8

INGREDIENTS

- 1 cup gluten-free all-purpose flour blend (we've used Arrowhead Mills Gluten Free All Purpose Baking Mix)
- 1 cup vegetable oil
- 1½ cups chopped yellow onion (about 1 large onion)
- 1 large green bell pepper, cored, seeded, and chopped (about 1 cup)
- 2 cloves garlic, crushed
- 1 pound gluten-free smoked sausage, such as andouille or kielbasa, sliced into bite-size rounds
- 2 teaspoons roughly chopped fresh thyme leaves
- 1 teaspoon celery salt
- ¼ teaspoon cayenne pepper, plus more if desired
- 3 bay leaves
- Black pepper to taste
- 6½ cups chicken stock or water
- 1 pound boneless, skinless chicken breasts, cut into bite-size chunks
- 1½ teaspoons Emeril's Rustic Rub or Original Essence Seasoning, or meat rub or Cajun seasoning of your choice
- ½ cup thinly sliced green onions (about 5 green onions)
- 2 tablespoons chopped fresh parsley
- Cooked white or brown rice, for serving

STEPS

1 In a large (8- to 10-quart) soup pot, combine the flour and oil over medium heat, stirring constantly and gently for 20 to 25 minutes, to make the roux.

2 Add the onion, bell pepper, and garlic to the pot. Stir and cook until the vegetables are slightly softened, about 5 minutes.

3 Add the sausage, thyme, celery salt, cayenne, bay leaves, and a bit of black pepper to the pot. Stir and cook for an additional 5 minutes.

4 Add the stock or water and stir until the roux mixture and liquid are well combined. Turn the heat to high and bring to a gentle boil.

5 Once the soup is boiling, turn the heat down to low and simmer uncovered for 1 hour, stirring frequently.

6 Meanwhile, place the chicken pieces in a bowl and sprinkle with the Rustic Rub or Essence Seasoning. Put aside in the refrigerator until needed.

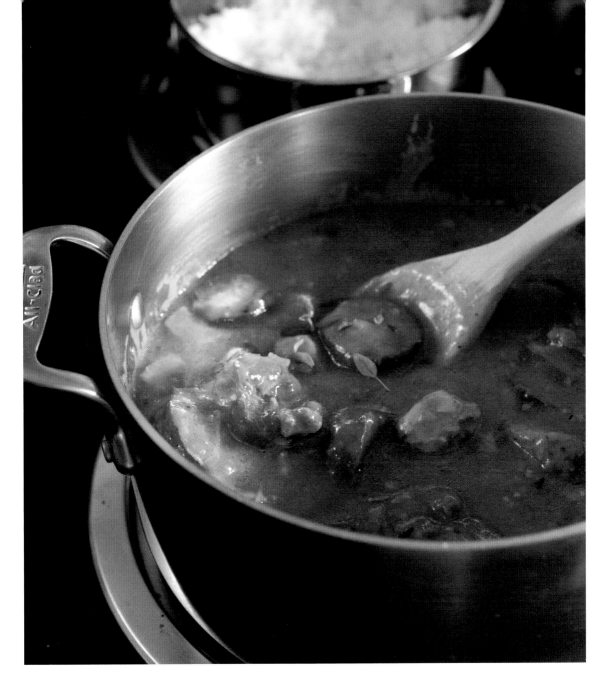

7 After the hour's cooking time is up, add the seasoned chicken to the pot and simmer uncovered for an additional 2 hours, stirring frequently and skimming off any fat that rises to the top.

8 Turn off the heat, remove the bay leaves, and stir in all but a tablespoon or so of the green onions and all the parsley.

9 Serve immediately in deep bowls, over the cooked rice of your choice and garnished with a sprinkling of the remaining green onions on top.

chunky corn chowder

INGREDIENTS

2 medium-size baking potatoes, peeled and diced (about 4 cups)

1 cup diced carrot

6 slices bacon, chopped

⅔ cup diced yellow onion

¼ cup gluten-free all-purpose flour blend (we've used Arrowhead Mills Gluten Free All Purpose Baking Mix)

1 teaspoon salt

¼ teaspoon black pepper

Pinch of cayenne pepper

3 cups milk

1 cup half-and-half

2 cups cooked fresh corn (from about 4 ears)

We grew up in New England, and chowder was a staple in our home and in many others. People historically favored fish or shellfish as the featured chowder ingredient, but corn replaces clams or oysters quite successfully in this delicious recipe, giving it a personality of its own. If we can, we love going to our local farmers' market to get freshly picked corn to use in this chowder. Or you can use your leftover corn from a barbecue or crab boil. Whatever the source, fresh corn really adds wonderful earthiness to this dish.

SERVES 4 TO 6

STEPS

❶ Combine the potatoes and carrot in a medium-size sauce-pan. Add water to cover and bring to a boil over medium-high heat. Cook until the vegetables are fork tender, about 10 to 15 minutes.

❷ While the veggies are cooking, fry the bacon in a medium-size saucepan over medium heat until crisp. Add the onion and sauté in the bacon grease until tender, 5 to 7 minutes.

❸ Blend in the flour blend, salt, black pepper, and cayenne pepper. Using a whisk, stir in the milk and half-and-half to blend well.

❹ When the potatoes and carrots are cooked, remove from the heat, drain, and add them to the mixture in the saucepan. Increase the heat to medium-high and bring the soup to a gentle boil. This will help it start to thicken.

❺ Once the boil is reached, turn the heat down to medium-low. Add the corn and cook just until it is heated through. Remove from the heat, taste and adjust the seasoning, and serve.

portuguese chourico
and peppers stew

INGREDIENTS

Salt

¾ pound small red potatoes, peeled and cut into bite-size chunks

1 pound chourico, or Spanish chorizo, cut into bite-size chunks, casings removed if possible

1 large yellow onion, halved and sliced

1 large green bell pepper, cored, seeded, and roughly sliced (about 2 cups)

2 cloves garlic, crushed

1½ teaspoons fresh thyme leaves, roughly chopped

1 teaspoon crushed red pepper flakes, plus more if desired

2 cans (14 ounces each) chopped tomatoes

1 can (14 ounces) lima beans, drained

3 tablespoons tomato paste

Pinch of smoked paprika

4 cups vegetable stock

We both grew up, for the most part, in a small town in southeastern Massachusetts. Somerset, like many towns in the area, is home to a sizable population of Portuguese Americans. In fact, we can think of only a few childhood friends or even family who weren't of Portuguese descent! We grew up eating a lot of meals that contained the spicy chourico, peppers, onions, and smoky paprika flavor profile. Just the smell of those flavors brings us right back to our childhood—memories of our grandmother Cabral's house and looking forward to a steaming bowl of soup or stew after playing outside on a cold winter's day. Try to use the best-quality chourico, or chorizo as it's also commonly spelled, that you can find. We always recommend removing the meat from the casing if possible. This really is a taste of our childhood, a rich and spicy dish worthy of its Portuguese heritage.

SERVES 4 TO 6

STEPS

1 In a large saucepan of boiling salted water, cook the potatoes until fork tender, about 13 to 15 minutes. Drain and set aside.

2 In a large (8-quart) stockpot over medium heat, fry the chourico for 3 to 4 minutes.

3 Add the onion, bell pepper, garlic, thyme, and crushed red pepper flakes and stir well. Cook another 5 minutes.

4 Add the tomatoes, drained lima beans, tomato paste, paprika, stock, and a pinch of salt. Stir well.

5 Cook over medium heat for 15 minutes

6 Add the potatoes, stir well, cover with a lid, and cook another 10 to 15 minutes.

7 Serve the soup in bowls along with your favorite gluten-free bread or rolls. We love Against The Grain Gourmet's gluten-free baguettes.

pumpkin *and* chili soup *with* autumnal spice

INGREDIENTS

2 tablespoons vegetable or olive oil

1 tablespoon lightly salted butter

1 medium-size yellow onion, chopped

2 cloves garlic, minced

1 teaspoon finely chopped fresh ginger

1 red chili pepper, seeded, deveined, and finely chopped

Salt to taste

1 small pumpkin (about 3¼ pounds), peeled, seeded, and cubed, or enough to make 5 cups

½ teaspoon ground nutmeg or a generous grating of fresh nutmeg

Black pepper to taste

5 cups vegetable stock or water

¾ cup half-and-half

Toasted pumpkin seeds, for garnish (optional)

Fresh chives, finely chopped or left whole, for garnish (optional)

Summers in Louisiana are famously hot, so you can imagine how much we look forward to fall, our favorite time of year. The cool nights, the football games, the sweaters. Then there are all the warm, hearty meals, such as this soup, which tastes like pure autumn in a bowl. With its deep orange color, Pumpkin and Chili Soup is a particularly beautiful dish, especially served with a sprinkle of roasted pumpkin seeds or parsnip crisps on top. For a delicious vegan option, just omit the butter and cream—all the autumnal yum will still be there for you. You could also substitute butternut squash, if desired. Try this at your next fall get-together or as a scrumptious addition to your Thanksgiving Day meal.

SERVES 6 TO 8

STEPS

1 In a medium-size (6-quart) stockpot, heat the oil and butter over medium heat. Add the onion, garlic, ginger, chili pepper, and a pinch of salt and sauté until the onion is slightly softened, about 5 minutes.

2 Add the pumpkin, nutmeg, and salt and pepper to taste and stir well.

3 Add the stock, turn the heat to medium high, and bring to a gentle boil. Cook for 8 minutes.

4 Turn the heat down to low and simmer uncovered for 30 minutes, stirring frequently.

5 Add the half-and-half, stir well, and taste for seasoning. You may want a bit more nutmeg for your liking. Turn off the heat.

6 If using a hand-held emulsion blender, you can blend the soup directly in the pot. If using a regular blender, allow the soup to cool slightly before blending in batches, using a puree setting if possible. (Hot liquids expand in a blender, so be sure to have a firm hand and a kitchen towel on the lid. You want to serve the soup, not wear it!)

7 After blending, serve the soup warm, garnished with a sprinkling of roasted pumpkin seeds and the chives, if desired.

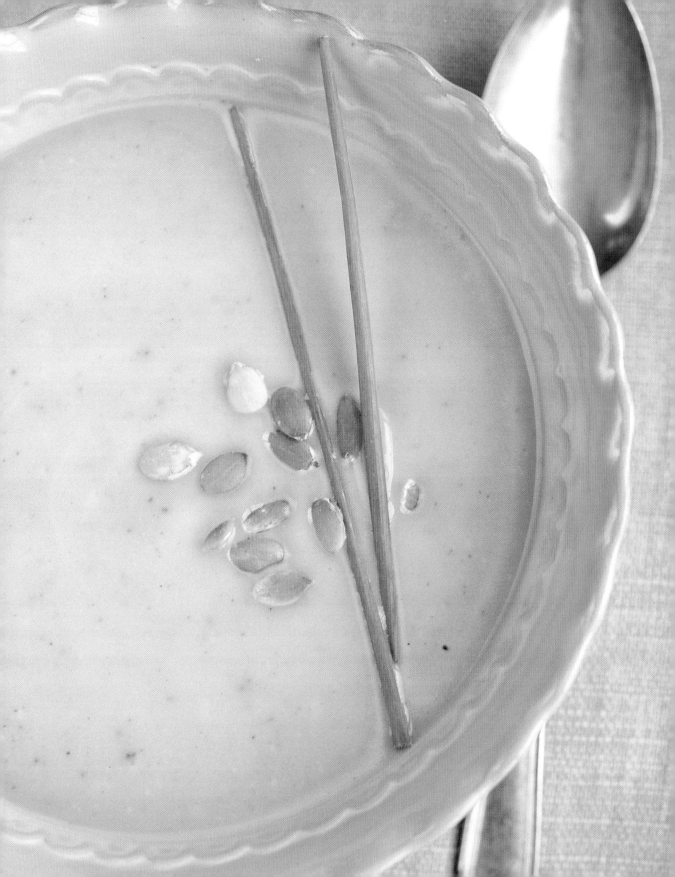

potato soup

INGREDIENTS

3 to 4 baking potatoes, peeled and chunked into similar-size pieces

10 slices bacon, diced

6 cups chicken stock

1 cup diced celery

1 cup diced yellow onion

¼ cup gluten-free all-purpose flour blend (we've used Arrowhead Mills Gluten Free All Purpose Baking Mix)

½ teaspoon salt

¼ teaspoon black pepper

Chives, sour cream, and grated cheddar, for garnish

Wonderfully dressed baked potatoes are high on many people's list of favorite foods, and our lists are no exception. This unique take on the baked potato brings the flavors of a fully dressed favorite spud in the form of a soup, one that is quite easy to make and can be served as either a starter or an entrée, depending on portion size. It also allows room for personalization. You can garnish the soup with any or all of your favorite potato toppings to create a soup as special as you are.

SERVES 6 TO 8

STEPS

❶ In a large saucepan of boiling salted water, cook the potatoes until tender, about 13 to 15 minutes. Drain and set aside.

❷ Fry the bacon in a medium-size (6-quart) stockpot over medium heat. When it is crispy, remove it from the pot with a slotted spoon and set aside.

❸ While the bacon is cooking, blend about three-quarters of the potatoes with 1 cup of the chicken stock in a blender. Set the blended mixture aside and reserve the remaining potatoes for use later.

❹ Add the celery and onion to the bacon grease in the pot and sauté for about 5 minutes.

❺ Add the flour blend, salt, and pepper to the vegetables in the pot to make a roux. Cook for 2 to 3 minutes, making sure to blend the flour with the other ingredients.

❻ Gradually add the remaining 5 cups chicken stock, stirring until the mixture begins to thicken.

❼ Once thickening begins to occur, add the blended potato mixture along with the reserved diced potatoes. Simmer uncovered for 10 to 15 minutes.

❽ Take off the heat and re-season as desired. Serve garnished with the reserved bacon, crumbled; chives; cheddar; and sour cream. Or add whatever your preferred toppings are and enjoy!

mushroom bisque

INGREDIENTS

2 tablespoons olive oil

1 pound cremini, or baby bella, mushrooms, brushed clean and sliced (about 6 cups)

½ cup chopped green onions

4 cups chicken or vegetable stock

6 tablespoons (¾ stick) unsalted butter

3 cups milk

⅓ cup gluten-free all-purpose flour blend (we've used Arrowhead Mills Gluten Free All Purpose Baking Mix)

1 cup heavy cream

2 tablespoons sherry

1½ teaspoons salt

15 drops Tabasco sauce

Black pepper to taste

Mushrooms tend to be like in-laws—you either love them or hate them. Mushrooms' rich, earthy flavors overpower some palates, while others enjoy almost every variety out there. This particular bisque lends itself to most any variety of mushroom, but we found it tasted best when we used cremini, or mini portobellos, called baby bellas. If you are feeling adventurous, try it out with a different type of mushroom and let us know how it comes out! As with many of our recipes, you can replace the chicken stock with vegetable stock if you are looking for a vegetarian option.

SERVES 6 TO 8

STEPS

❶ In a large skillet heat the olive oil over medium heat. Add the mushrooms and green onions and sauté for about 5 minutes, or until the mushrooms are tender.

❷ Transfer the mushrooms and green onions to a blender along with the chicken or vegetable stock and process until the mixture is smooth. Set aside.

❸ In a medium-size saucepan melt the butter. Simultaneously, in a separate saucepan heat the milk. Once the butter is completely melted, stir in the flour blend and cook for 1 to 3 minutes.

❹ Once the flour blend and butter are combined, add the hot milk. Whisk the mixture until it is smooth and begins to thicken.

❺ Add the cream, sherry, blended mushroom mixture, salt, Tabasco, and black pepper to taste. Bring to a simmer. Remove from the heat and serve.

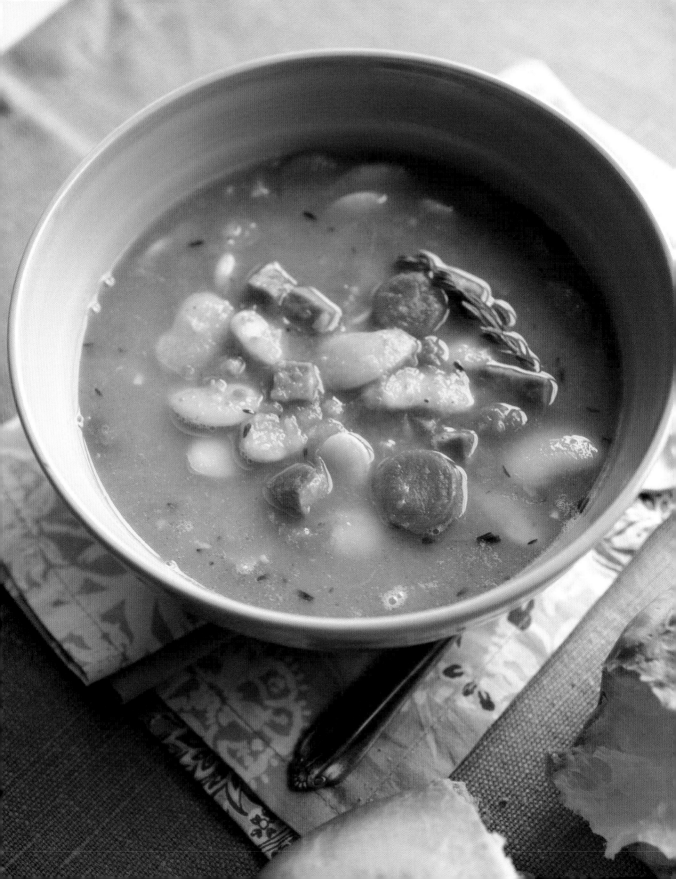

hearty lima bean *and* ham soup

INGREDIENTS

1 pound dried large lima beans, soaked for at least 2 hours in water

2 tablespoons olive oil

1 tablespoon unsalted butter

1½ cups chopped carrot (about 3 medium-size carrots, peeled)

¾ cup chopped celery

1 cup chopped yellow onion

1 clove garlic, minced

1 pound uncured ham steak, cubed

Salt and black pepper to taste

8 cups vegetable stock

2 cups water

1 bay leaf

1 tablespoon fresh thyme leaves

Sour cream or crème fraîche, for garnish (optional)

Jilly came up with this recipe for her amazing brother-in-law, Steve (aka Stevarino), who has an unabashed love for American staples like ham, carrots, and, yes, soft, creamy, and oh-so-filling lima beans. He deemed this creation "the hibernation soup" because just one bowlful is hearty enough to see you through until next winter! This is a wonderfully simple soup to make on a cold winter's day, and it makes a large enough batch that you could always freeze half. For a vegetarian option, you could omit the ham and simply double the amounts of carrots and celery. Either way, this soup is packed with heart-healthy fiber and protein. In honor of Steve, let us all hail the mighty lima bean!

SERVES 8 TO 10

STEPS

1 Drain the soaked beans and set aside.

2 In a large (8-quart) stockpot, heat the oil and butter over medium heat. Add the carrots, celery, onion, and garlic and sauté, stirring occasionally, until the vegetables start to soften slightly, about 5 minutes.

3 Add the ham with a bit of salt and pepper, stir well, and sauté another 5 minutes.

4 Add the beans, stock, water, and bay leaf to the pot and stir well.

5 Increase the heat to medium high and bring to a boil. Cook uncovered for 15 minutes.

6 Turn the heat to medium low and skim off any fat that rises to the top. Add the thyme leaves and stir well. Cover and simmer for 1 hour, or until the beans are cooked through, stirring occasionally. If the 10 cups of liquid are absorbed before the beans have sufficiently cooked, you can add 1 to 2 cups of water.

7 When ready to serve, remove the bay leaf. Taste the soup and re-season if needed. Ladle into bowls, topping each serving with a spoonful of sour cream or crème fraîche, if desired.

fresh tomato basil soup

INGREDIENTS

3 pounds ripe tomatoes

2 tablespoons olive oil

2 teaspoons minced garlic

2 medium-size yellow onions, coarsely chopped (about 2 cups)

1⅓ cups chicken or vegetable stock

⅓ cup coarsely chopped fresh basil leaves

½ teaspoon salt

¼ teaspoon black pepper

This surprisingly light and tasty soup works two ways: served hot in the winter or just barely warmed in the summer. One way or the other, it does require the tomatoes to be peeled before preparing. Some very skilled individuals might be able to peel a tomato by hand. If you are like us, however, you will need to follow the steps below to blanch your tomatoes and facilitate easier peeling. To get the perfect texture, we found that it's best to use a blender or hand emulsifier instead of a food processor to blend the soup. It comes out creamier that way.

SERVES 4 TO 6

STEPS

❶ To begin, you must first blanch the tomatoes so you can peel them easily. Bring water to a boil in a large (8-quart) stockpot. Use enough water so the tomatoes can be totally immersed. Score the bottom (nonstem) side of each tomato with an X. Once the water is boiling, carefully add the tomatoes and boil for 2 to 3 minutes. Immediately drain the pot and run cold water over the tomatoes for a few minutes, until they are cool enough to handle.

❷ Once the tomatoes are manageable, gently remove and discard the skins. Seed the tomatoes and chop the flesh. Set the flesh aside.

❸ In a medium-size (6-quart) stockpot over medium heat, heat the olive oil. Add the onions and garlic and sauté for 5 to 7 minutes, or until the onions are tender.

❹ Add the tomatoes, chicken or vegetable stock, basil, salt, and pepper and simmer uncovered until the tomatoes are covered with liquid, about 25 to 30 minutes. Stir occasionally so the tomatoes don't burn on the bottom of the pan.

❺ Carefully pour the hot soup mixture into a blender. Process on high until the texture is smooth and no lumps remain. If the entire amount doesn't fit into your blender, blend the soup in batches and then recombine. If you are using a hand emulsifier, you can emulsify the soup in the same pot or transfer it to a different bowl. (Just be careful not to splash the hot liquid up onto yourself…ouch!)

❻ Re-season if necessary. Either serve immediately or let the soup cool and then serve.

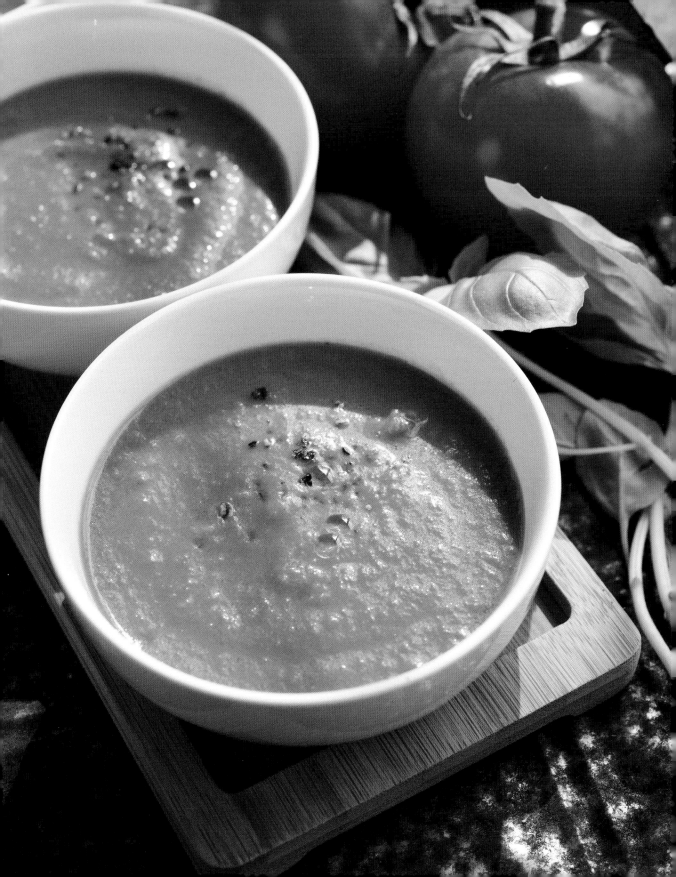

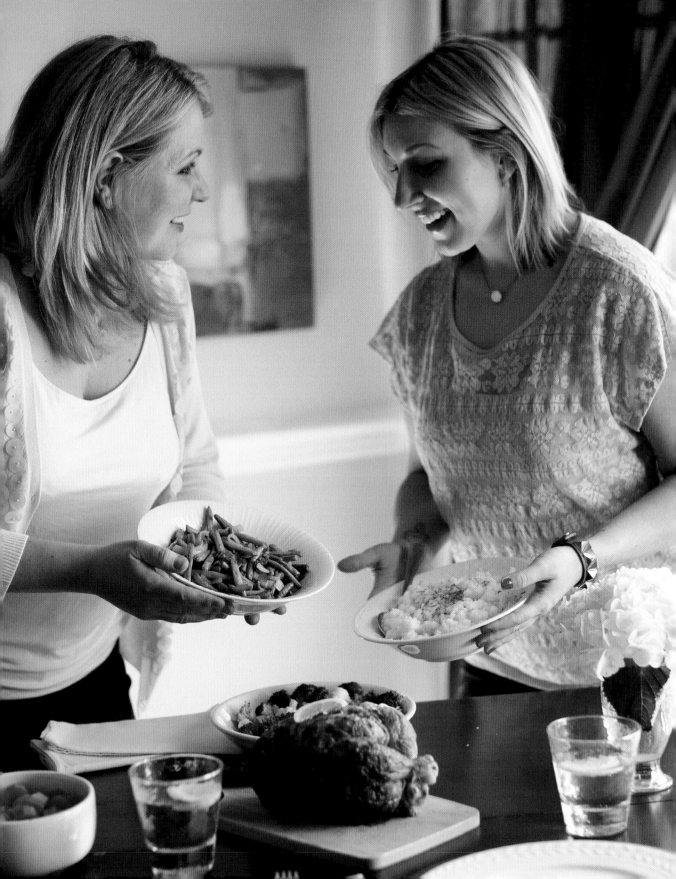

sides

Growing up, we have to admit that the foods that accompanied our entrée were usually more desirable to us than the entrée itself. And, typically, we preferred carbs, carbs, and more carbs in the form of gluten-laden breads and pastas. One of the most difficult adjustments we had to make after we were diagnosed as gluten intolerant was changing the side dishes we relied on, craved, and loved. It was a *long*, slow journey, but after a lot of trial and error, we managed to replicate gluten-free versions of most of our favorites. We were also surprised to find a previously unknown fondness for vegetables!

In this chapter, you'll find our tweaked versions of old favorites like mac and cheese and cornbread. You'll also find our new favorites, like Cheesy Shrimp and Crab Grits and Crumby Garlic Green Beans. Whether you are looking for the perfect accompaniment to a chicken entrée or a vegetarian tofu dish, there is a perfectly suited side dish (or two!) somewhere in this list. Have fun finding your favorite!

jalapeño *and* cheddar cornbread

1 tablespoon unsalted butter, plus additional for topping

1 cup gluten-free all-purpose flour blend (we've used Arrowhead Mills Gluten Free All Purpose Baking Mix)

1 cup finely ground cornmeal

1 tablespoon granulated sugar

2 teaspoons gluten-free baking powder

2 teaspoons salt

½ teaspoon baking soda

⅔ cup buttermilk

2 large eggs plus 1 large egg white, lightly beaten

1 cup grated cheddar cheese

½ cup canned creamed corn

3 small green onions, thinly sliced

2 to 3 jalapeño chilies, seeded, deveined, and finely chopped

Cornbread is a Southern staple and makes the perfect partner to any meal. Add in the spice of the jalapeños and the savory cheddar cheese and you have a cornbread that dreams are made of. True to Southern tradition, we usually use a large cast-iron skillet to make our cornbread. But, if you don't have one, this works just as well baked in an 8 × 8–inch baking dish. Feel free to add as many jalapeños as you and your taste buds can handle. Jilly often serves this at brunch, drizzled with a bit of maple syrup and presented alongside eggs and bacon. Yum! So shake things up and try this gluten-free cornbread for breakfast, lunch, or dinner.

SERVES 6 TO 8

STEPS

❶ Preheat the oven to 400°F.

❷ In a cast-iron skillet over medium-low heat, melt the 1 tablespoon butter. If using an 8 × 8–inch baking dish instead, simply grease the bottom of the dish with some of the butter and place the remainder in the bottom of the dish. Set the skillet or dish aside.

❸ Sift the flour blend, cornmeal, sugar, baking powder, salt, and baking soda together into a large bowl.

❹ In a small bowl mix the buttermilk and eggs together well.

❺ Fold the wet ingredients into the dry ingredients to thoroughly mix.

❻ Fold in the cheese, creamed corn, green onions, and chilies, and stir until well combined.

❼ Pour the mixture into the prepared skillet or baking dish and dab a bit more butter on top.

❽ Bake for 30 to 35 minutes, or until a toothpick inserted in the center comes out clean and the top is golden brown.

❾ Leave to cool in the pan or dish for a few minutes before slicing and serving while warm.

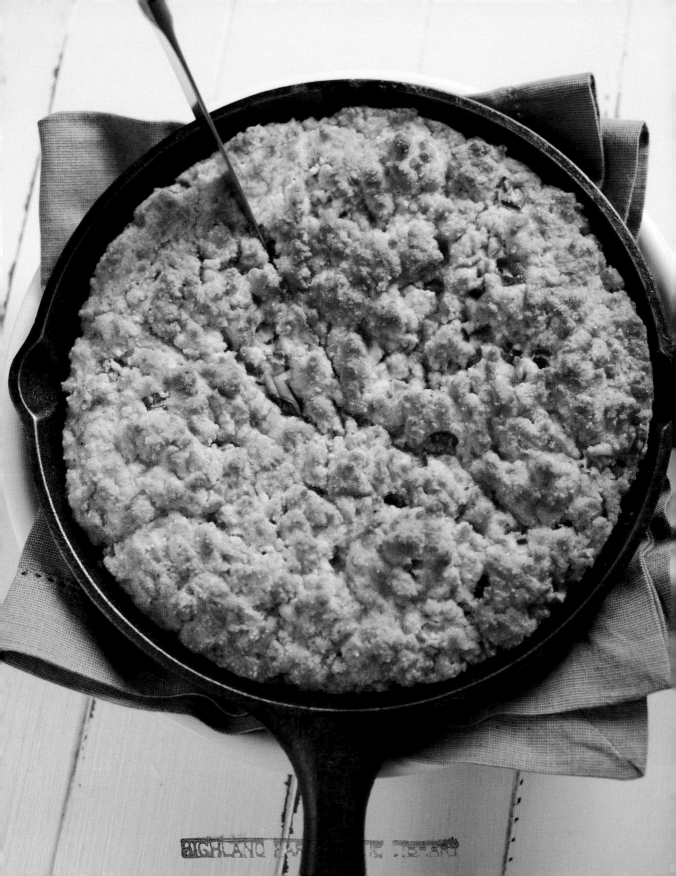

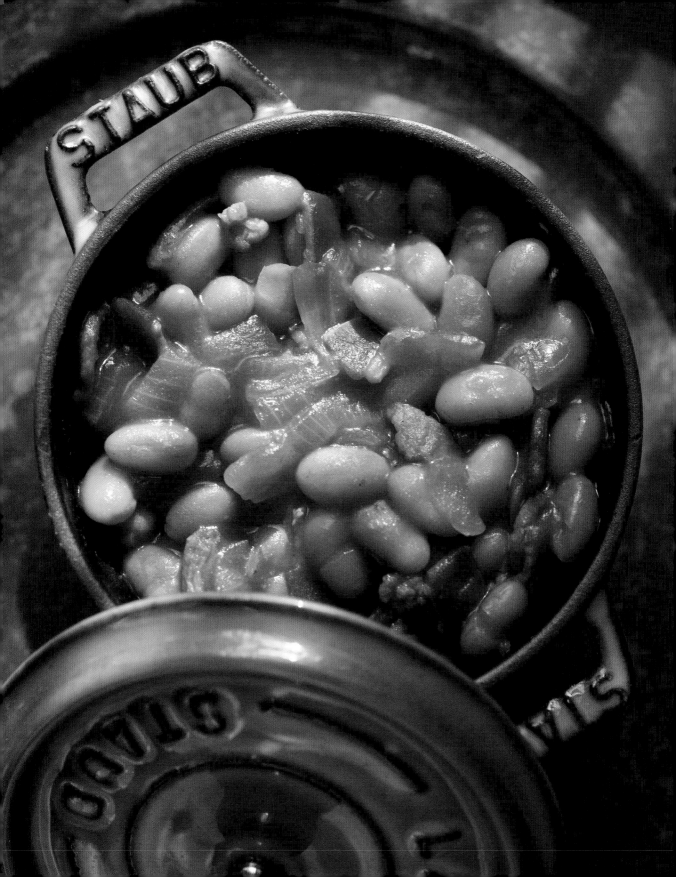

baked beans

INGREDIENTS

4 slices bacon, chopped

2/3 cup diced yellow onion

1/3 cup ketchup

3 tablespoons (packed) light brown sugar

3 tablespoons chicken stock or water

1 tablespoon molasses

2 teaspoons gluten-free Worcestershire sauce (we like Lea & Perrins)

1 teaspoon dry mustard

1/4 teaspoon minced garlic

1 can (15 ounces) navy beans, drained

Growing up, we could always count on baked beans at family reunions, barbecues, and Fourth of July parties. However, looking back, we realize we were probably eating the canned version the whole time… not that there is anything wrong with that, but this made-from-scratch alternative is so easy to make, even the most die-hard Bush's Baked Beans fan may convert. They're super sweet and smoky, a humid summer evening in a bowl. If you want to make them for a group, just double or triple the recipe and use a larger baking dish.

SERVES 4

STEPS

❶ Preheat the oven to 350°F.

❷ In a medium-size skillet, cook the bacon over medium-high heat until crispy. Remove the bacon pieces with a slotted spoon and drain all but about 1 teaspoon of bacon grease from the skillet. Sauté the onion in the remaining grease over medium-high heat until tender, about 3 to 5 minutes.

❸ In a large bowl mix together all the ingredients except the beans. The mixture should be of a uniform consistency and sort of syrupy.

❹ Once the mixture is the correct consistency, fold in the beans and mix gently but thoroughly. Pour the mixture into a small baking dish, cover, and bake for 20 minutes. Remove the cover and bake another 20 minutes.

❺ Remove the beans from the oven and serve.

collard greens

1 tablespoon olive oil

1 cup sliced onion

2 teaspoons minced garlic

1 large head collard greens, washed, deribbed, and roughly chopped (about 8 to 10 cups)

½ pound ham hock

½ pound cooked ham, diced

4 cups chicken stock

⅛ teaspoon cayenne pepper

Salt to taste

This is our version of a wonderful Southern tradition. Southerners incorporate collard greens into all kinds of recipes, but our favorite is when they're served alone as a savory side. When we traveled outside of New Orleans, we were shocked to discover that many people, especially those up North, had never even heard of collard greens. Done right, collard greens should look fully limp and create a natural broth that's savory and smoky. The ham hock adds a distinctive flavor to these collards, so be sure to ask your butcher for one if you don't find it on the regular meat shelves. Butchers usually have some in back. Also, some people prefer to break the ham hock meat off the bone and incorporate it in the mixture once cooking is complete. Others prefer to simply remove the hock and serve the greens that way. Try it both ways to see which you prefer!

These greens take a while to cook, but they are certainly worth it! They are also known to be full of an array of vitamins and nutrients, an additional plus. Because the ham hock and the ham may already contain salt, wait until the greens are thoroughly cooked before seasoning with additional salt.

SERVES 4

STEPS

1 In a medium-size (6-quart) stockpot over medium heat, heat the olive oil. Add the onions and garlic and sauté for 5 to 7 minutes, or until the onions become tender.

2 Add all the other ingredients except the salt and simmer over medium-low heat for 1½ to 2 hours, or until the greens have become soft and almost soupy.

3 Adjust the seasoning as necessary and add salt at this point if needed. Either remove the hock whole or break off the meat into the greens before removing the bone. Stir until incorporated. Serve.

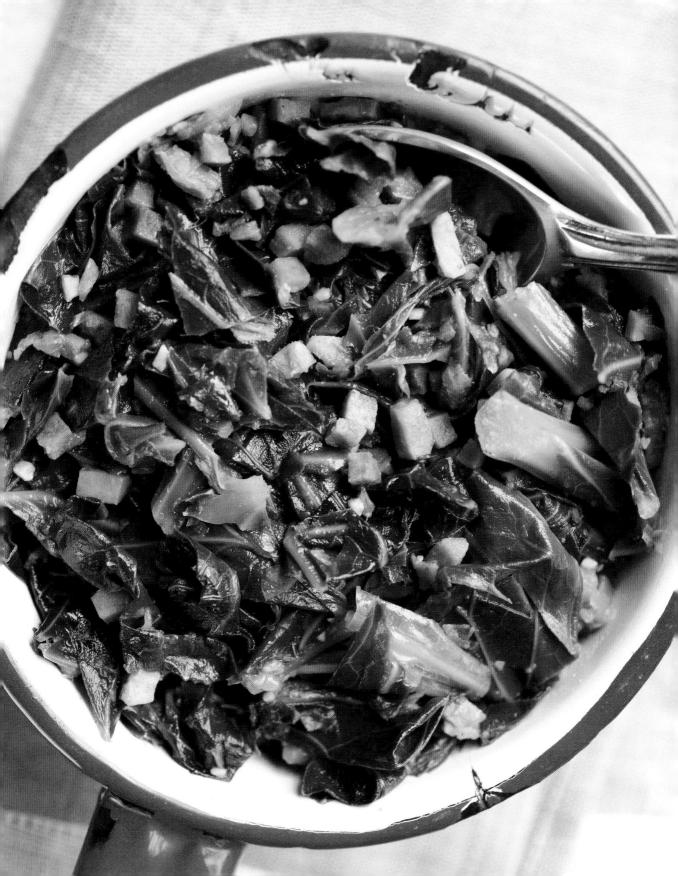

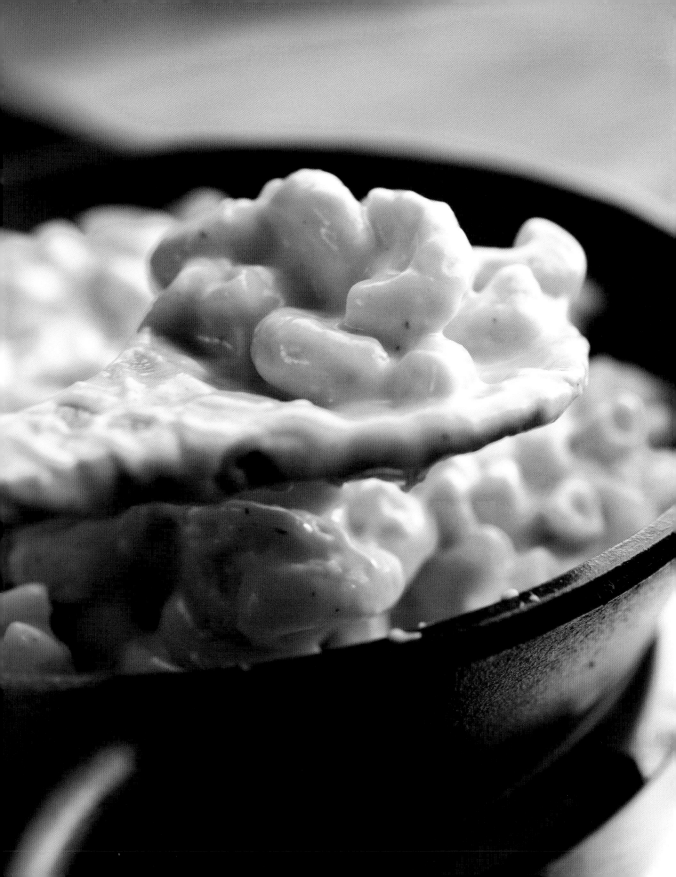

baked macaroni *and* cheese

INGREDIENTS

2 tablespoons unsalted butter

2 tablespoons gluten-free all-purpose flour blend (we've used Arrowhead Mills Gluten Free All Purpose Baking Mix)

2 cups milk

2¼ cups grated sharp cheddar cheese

½ teaspoon salt

¼ teaspoon black pepper

2 cups gluten-free macaroni, cooked al dente and drained

Everyone seems to have a signature macaroni recipe: macaroni with a fancy cheese or a crumb topping, seven-cheese macaroni, macaroni with different kinds of noodles—the list goes on and on. In our opinion, you really can't mess up any kind of noodle covered in creamy, melty cheese, but there is something particularly irresistible about this tried-and-true classic. We tried several variations of this to make sure the temperature and time were just perfect, so the macaroni is gooey on the inside but still stays together. While we like ours moderately seasoned, you can vary the salt and pepper to your liking. You can also prepare the whole dish a day in advance of baking if that's more convenient.

SERVES 6 TO 8

STEPS

1 Preheat the oven to 350°F.

2 In a large saucepan over medium-low heat, melt the butter. Whisk in the flour blend and cook, whisking constantly, for about 3 to 4 minutes.

3 Gradually whisk in the milk. Simmer, stirring frequently, for 10 to 15 minutes, or until the mixture is thick enough to coat a wooden spoon. The mixture will thicken as it cooks, so be sure to keep stirring it.

4 Remove from the heat and stir in 1½ cups of the cheese and the salt and pepper. Mix until the cheese is fully melted.

5 Stir the cooked macaroni into the cheese mixture.

6 Pour half of the resulting mixture into an 8 × 8–inch baking dish. Sprinkle evenly with half the remaining cheese. Pour in the rest of the macaroni mixture and finish with the remaining cheese.

7 Bake for about 30 minutes, or until the cheese on top starts to brown.

8 Remove from the oven, let sit for 5 minutes, and then serve.

crumby garlic green beans

INGREDIENTS

- 2 slices gluten-free bread, torn into large pieces
- 1 tablespoon unsalted butter
- 3 tablespoons freshly grated Parmesan cheese
- Salt and black pepper to taste
- 1 tablespoon minced garlic
- 2 tablespoons olive oil
- 2 teaspoons gluten-free all-purpose flour blend (we've used Arrowhead Mills Gluten Free All Purpose Baking Mix)
- 1 teaspoon minced fresh thyme leaves
- Pinch of crushed red pepper flakes
- 2 pounds green beans, ends trimmed
- ⅔ cup chicken stock
- 1 tablespoon lemon juice

Believe it or not, Jessie's son Jude looks forward to getting to eat green beans with his dinner. While he likes his perfectly plain, as nature intended, most of us need to add something to make them more appealing. And what better, more universally delicious ingredients to add than garlic, cheese, and bread! This neat recipe uses seasoned gluten-free bread crumbs to give the dish a distinct crunch, and takes the simple green bean to another level of addictiveness. You'll never serve plain salt-and-pepper green beans again.

SERVES 6 TO 8

STEPS

1 Grind the bread pieces in a food processor until coarse crumbs are formed. You want approximately 1⅓ to 1½ cups crumbs.

2 Melt the butter in a medium-size skillet over medium heat. Add the bread crumbs and sauté, stirring frequently, until the crumbs toast and become crunchy. This should take about 3 to 5 minutes.

3 Pour the crumbs into a bowl and toss with the cheese, a pinch of black pepper, and a pinch of salt. Set aside.

4 In the same skillet, sauté the garlic in the olive oil for 1 to 3 minutes over medium heat. Stir in the flour blend, thyme, and crushed red pepper flakes until well incorporated.

5 Add the green beans and chicken stock, stirring until the stock is evenly incorporated into the flour mixture. Cover and cook until the beans are soft on the outside but still crisp in the middle, about 4 to 6 minutes. Uncover and cook another 2 to 4 minutes.

6 Once the beans are of the desired tenderness, remove from the heat, stir in the lemon juice, and adjust the salt and pepper as desired.

7 Transfer to plates or a large serving dish and sprinkle the bread crumbs on top to serve.

portobello grits

1 cup instant grits

Chicken stock for cooking the grits (about 4 cups, depending on the brand of grits)

1 tablespoon unsalted butter

1 cup diced onion (We prefer Vidalia here, but any sweet onion will suffice.)

2 medium-size portobello mushroom caps, brushed clean and chopped (about 2½ cups)

2 teaspoons minced garlic

½ teaspoon salt

¼ teaspoon black pepper

⅓ cup freshly grated Parmesan cheese

¼ cup freshly grated Pecorino Romano cheese

These grits are an absolute hit every time we make them. The dish is similar to a risotto, but using corn grits instead of rice, equally delicious though slightly less filling (depending on how much you eat!), and less time consuming. The mushrooms combined with the cheesiness are truly scrumptious, a flavor combination that wows every single time. If you don't like portobello mushrooms, you can substitute the mushroom of your choice and the recipe will still be delicious!

Also, just in case you heard that line from the movie *My Cousin Vinny*, "No self respectin' Southerner uses instant grits"—we assure you, it isn't true. Sometimes even self-respecting Southerners are pressed for time! Because there are many kinds of instant grits, the recipe here is not specific about the amount of chicken stock to use. Just follow the recipe on the grits box for preparing the grits, but substitute chicken stock for the water.

SERVES 6 TO 8

STEPS

❶ In a medium-size saucepan, cook the grits according to package directions, replacing water with chicken stock.

❷ While the grits are cooking, melt the butter in a large skillet over medium-high heat. Add the onion and sauté, stirring frequently, for 5 to 10 minutes, or until the onion is soft and golden brown.

❸ Add the mushrooms, garlic, salt, and pepper and cook for another 5 minutes, or until the mushrooms are soft. Remove from the heat.

❹ When the grits are ready, stir in the mushroom mixture, along with the cheeses. Re-season as necessary and serve immediately.

cheesy shrimp *and* crab grits

INGREDIENTS

1 cup grits

1 cup grated cheddar cheese

1 cup freshly grated Parmesan cheese

3 tablespoons unsalted butter

½ teaspoon salt, plus more to taste

Cayenne pepper to taste

6 slices bacon, diced

2 cups sliced mushrooms (about 4 ounces, brushed clean)

1½ cups green onions, chopped

1 tablespoon minced garlic

1 pound shrimp, peeled and deveined

3 tablespoons chopped fresh parsley

1 cup lump crabmeat, picked over for shells (about 8 ounces)

Black pepper to taste

Grits have been a staple in Southern homes for generations. Made from corn, grits are an affordable and versatile component of traditional breakfast fare, although hearty, rich grits such as the ones here are best eaten with dinner. Of course, it didn't take many generations for someone to marry grits with another Cajun love, seafood! In Louisiana, shrimp and crab show up in lots of recipes, but this scrumptious side dish may be the best of them all. We've added creamy cheddar cheese and mushrooms to make it even more tempting. It does require plenty of salt, but make sure you taste as you sprinkle, so you don't go overboard!

SERVES 6

STEPS

❶ In a medium-size saucepan, cook the grits according to package directions. Once the grains are tender, remove from the heat and stir in the cheeses, butter, ½ teaspoon salt, and a pinch of cayenne. Set aside.

❷ In a medium-size skillet over medium heat, cook the bacon until it is crispy. Add the mushrooms, green onions, and garlic and sauté for 2 to 4 minutes, until the mushrooms begin to soften.

❸ Add the shrimp and parsley and cook until the color of the shrimp changes to pink, about 3 to 5 minutes, depending on the size of the shrimp.

❹ Pour the shrimp mixture into the saucepan with the grits. Add the crabmeat and fold everything together gently.

❺ Re-season with salt, cayenne, and black pepper as desired. Serve immediately.

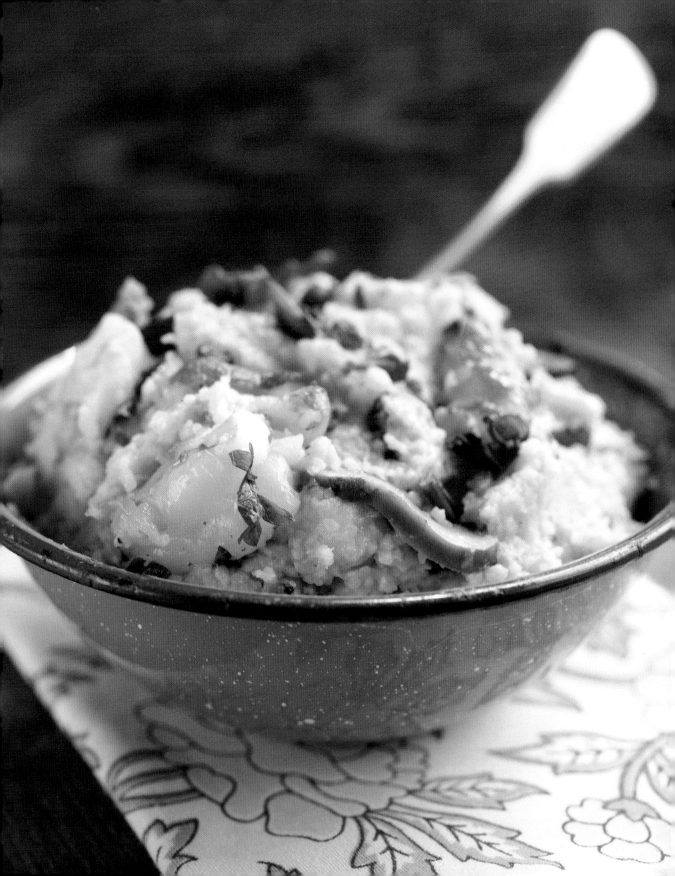

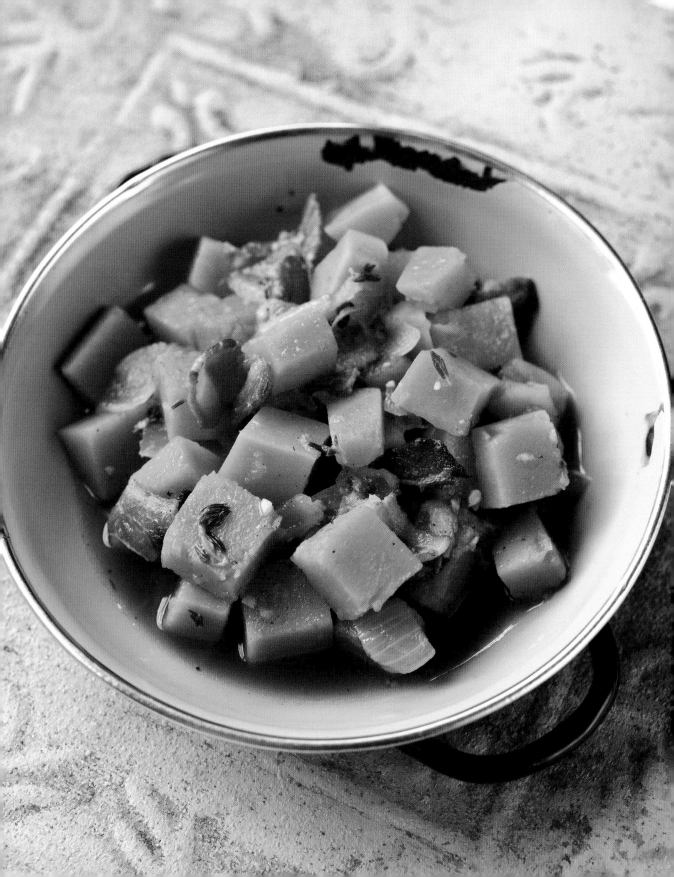

stewed butternut squash
with apples *and* smoked bacon

INGREDIENTS

4 strips thick-cut smoked bacon, diced

1½ cups small-diced onion

1 tablespoon minced garlic

2 tablespoons unsalted butter

1 Granny Smith apple, peeled, cored, and diced

1 butternut squash (2 pounds), peeled, seeds removed, and diced

¼ teaspoon freshly grated nutmeg

1 tablespoon chopped fresh thyme

1½ teaspoons salt

½ teaspoon freshly ground black pepper

¼ cup maple syrup

2 cups chicken stock

Butternut squash tends to be one of those vegetables some people are always hesitant to try to cook. Whether it is because they don't know what to do with it or just because it is kind of cumbersome to handle, this humble squash is seriously underrated. For this recipe, tart apples and smoky bacon combine with nutmeg, thyme, and maple syrup to produce a butternut squash dish that is flavorful, filling, and satisfying. Enjoy!

SERVES 6

STEPS

1 Set a medium-size sauté pan over medium heat. Add the bacon to the pan and render, stirring often, until crispy, 6 to 8 minutes.

2 Add the onion to the pan and cook until lightly caramelized, 4 to 5 minutes.

3 Add the garlic, butter, and apple to the pan and cook, stirring often, until the apple is tender, about 5 minutes.

4 Add the squash to the pan and increase the heat to medium-high. Cook the squash, undisturbed, for 3 to 4 minutes. Stir, and then add the nutmeg, thyme, salt, and pepper.

5 Cook for another 3 to 4 minutes and add the maple syrup and the stock. Bring the liquid to a boil, cover the pan, and reduce the heat to medium. Cook until the squash is tender and most of the liquid has evaporated, about 15 minutes.

6 Remove the lid, stir the squash gently, and re-season if necessary. Serve immediately, while hot.

green beans *with* bacon *and* onions

INGREDIENTS

1 pound green beans, ends trimmed

½ pound bacon, chopped

1 large yellow onion, halved lengthwise and sliced crosswise (about 2 cups)

Salt and black pepper to taste

Everything is better with bacon, right? We certainly think so, and these tasty beans prove it. The dish pairs well with lots of entrées, but we like them most served next to a nice, juicy filet and a fully dressed baked potato. Yum! For those of you who might prefer a bacon-less option (are there really any of you out there, now, come on!), you can always substitute some olive oil for the bacon fat. We also find it helpful to cook the beans in a large skillet with a lip so they don't escape onto the stovetop as you stir them.

SERVES 4

STEPS

1 Prepare a large bowl of ice water.

2 Blanch the beans in a saucepan of boiling water until they start to soften—maybe 2 to 3 minutes at most. Drain the beans and place them in the ice-water bath to shock them, drain again, and set aside.

3 In a large skillet over medium heat, cook the chopped bacon until it is crispy. Leaving the bacon in the skillet, drain off all but 1 to 2 tablespoons of the grease.

4 To the skillet add the onion and beans along with salt and pepper to your liking. Stir to incorporate all the ingredients. Continue to sauté until the onion is translucent and soft.

5 Remove from the heat and serve immediately.

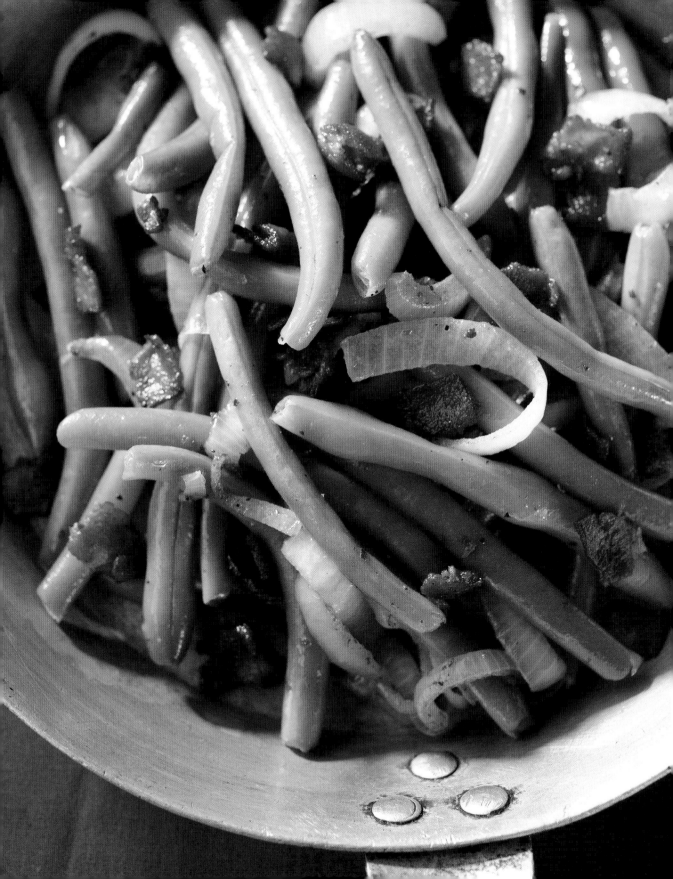

pancetta *and* sage potato pie

INGREDIENTS

4 ounces good-quality pancetta, roughly chopped

2 tablespoons unsalted butter

2 medium-size yellow onions, halved lengthwise and thinly sliced crosswise (about 4 cups)

3 cloves garlic, crushed

2 heaping tablespoons fresh sage leaves, roughly chopped

Salt and black pepper to taste

2½ pounds red-skinned potatoes, scrubbed well and thinly sliced, using a mandoline or sharp knife

1 tablespoon Emeril's Original Essence Seasoning or Cajun seasoning of your choice

1⅔ cups heavy cream

Chives, for garnish (optional)

What a decadent side dish this potato pie makes! Who knew the humble potato could be so elegant? We must warn you that this is quite a heavy dish, due to the cream and butter. But in our eyes that makes it all the more suited for a special occasion! This is an impressive dish to serve as a holiday accompaniment that you can make ahead of time and simply reheat. We recommend making this in a 13 × 9–inch baking dish. Once you slice into this pie, the layers are so enticing that you should be prepared for people to bow to your culinary skills. And trust us, it's worth the extra time on the treadmill.

SERVES 6 TO 8

STEPS

1 Preheat the oven to 400°F.

2 Lightly grease a 13 × 9–inch baking dish and set aside.

3 In a medium-size sauté pan over medium heat, fry the pancetta in 1 tablespoon of the butter until crispy, about 2 to 3 minutes.

4 Add the onions, garlic, and sage leaves and stir well to make sure everything is coated with the butter and pancetta grease.

5 Season with salt and pepper to taste and sauté until the onion is slightly softened, about another 5 minutes.

6 Remove from the heat and set aside.

7 Place a single layer of potato slices along the bottom and up the sides of the prepared baking dish, making sure to slightly overlap the slices on the bottom, until the bottom of the dish is fully covered. This will create your "crust." (You should have enough potatoes left to make three more layers.)

8 Season the potatoes in the dish with a bit of the Essence Seasoning.

9 Spoon one-third of the pancetta and onion mixture over the bottom layer of potatoes.

10 Sprinkle the pancetta-and-onion layer with a bit of pepper and add enough cream to moisten and cover that layer along with whatever potatoes are still visible.

11 Repeat steps 7 to 10 twice: layer of potatoes, Essence Seasoning, pancetta-onion mixture, and cream.

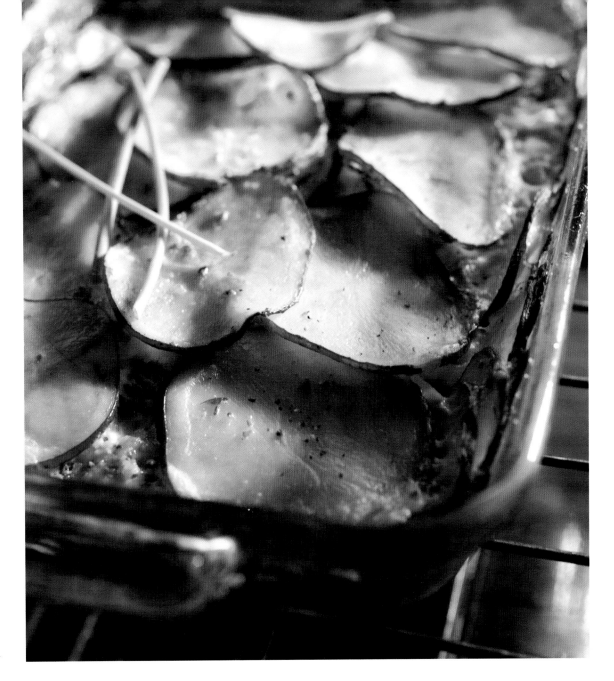

⑫ Make a final layer of potatoes and sprinkle Essence Seasoning on top. Ideally, the top layer should be level with the potatoes around the sides, but it's okay if it's not.

⑬ Dot with the remaining 1 tablespoon butter and cover loosely with foil.

⑭ Place on a baking tray and bake for 45 minutes. Remove the foil and bake another 35 to 45 minutes. You want the potatoes to be soft and tender and the top bubbly and golden brown.

⑮ Let the pie cool slightly. Garnish with whole chives, if desired, and serve.

sour cream *and* chive mash

INGREDIENTS

Salt

6 small to medium potatoes, Idaho or creamer variety, peeled, halved, and cut into chunks

½ cup sour cream

½ cup milk or cream, any % fat you prefer

⅓ cup finely chopped fresh chives

2 cloves garlic, crushed

½ teaspoon celery salt

Black pepper to taste

All the years Jilly has lived in London, England, have forced her to master the art of making a great mashed potato, or "mash," as it's known. This recipe had to be tried, tasted, and tested many times before we both deemed it cookbook worthy. We've noticed that people have very strong opinions when it comes to the consistency of their mash. Some people like theirs with lumps; some prefer a thicker or more moist variety. Whatever your preference, we think we've got even the pickiest of mash connoisseurs covered with our version. Give it a try for yourself and see.

SERVES 4

STEPS

❶ In a large saucepan of boiling salted water, cook the potatoes until they are almost falling apart, about 20 minutes.

❷ Drain the potatoes and return to the pan.

❸ Add the sour cream and milk or cream. Mash, using a masher, until you reach your desired consistency. You can always add more milk if you like your mash creamier than the results here.

❹ Stir in the chopped chives, garlic, celery salt, and a bit of salt and pepper to taste, mixing well to incorporate all the seasonings.

❺ Serve immediately, while still warm.

balsamic-glazed asparagus

INGREDIENTS

2 pounds asparagus

½ cup balsamic vinegar

¼ cup plus 2 tablespoons
extra virgin olive oil

Salt and black pepper to taste

¼ cup freshly grated
Parmesan cheese

For Jessie, one surprising result of discovering her gluten intolerance was developing more of a taste for vegetables than ever before. Maybe it was because she could no longer fill up on her favorite starches, or perhaps having to scrutinize labels made her more vigilant about what she put in her body. Nevertheless, asparagus is one of those vegetables Jessie once avoided but now really enjoys, both for their beautiful presentation and for their unique grassy taste. The balsamic glaze here adds a new twist to the usual garlic- or lemon-spiked preparation. We prefer the asparagus cooked slightly al dente, but you can boil them for a little bit less or more time depending on your crunch preference. Be sure to trim the tough ends off before you cook and eat the asparagus, though…yuck!

SERVES 4 TO 6

STEPS

❶ Preheat the oven to 350°F.

❷ After trimming the tough ends off the asparagus, cook them in a large saucepan of boiling water until slightly crunchy, 3 to 5 minutes, depending on the thickness of the asparagus spears. Remove from the heat, drain, and arrange in an 8 × 8–inch baking dish. Set aside.

❸ To make the glaze, whisk together the balsamic vinegar and the ¼ cup of olive oil.

❹ Drizzle the remaining 2 tablespoons olive oil over the asparagus, tossing the asparagus gently to coat, and season with salt and pepper. Pour the glaze over the asparagus and sprinkle evenly with the grated Parmesan.

❺ Bake for 5 to 10 minutes, or until the cheese has melted and is lightly browned. Serve immediately.

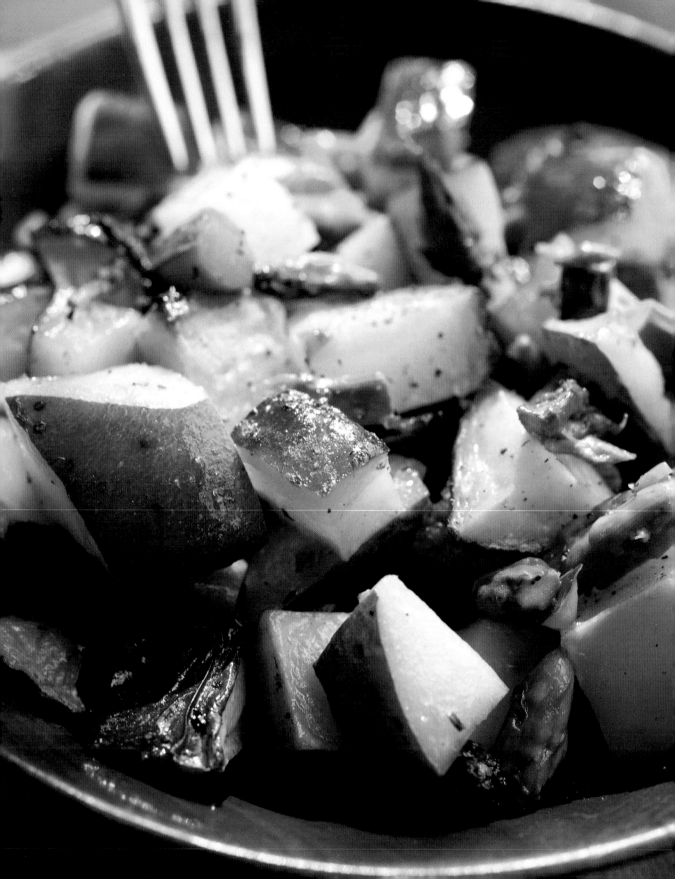

roasted asparagus *and* potatoes

INGREDIENTS

1 bunch asparagus, tough ends trimmed

2 to 4 tablespoons olive oil

4 medium-size red potatoes, scrubbed and cubed (about 2 cups)

½ teaspoon salt

¼ teaspoon black pepper

This simple dish is a snap to make, tastes great, and is great for you. It's a starch and veggie all in one! Depending on your affinity for olive oil, you may use as little as 2 tablespoons or as much as ¼ cup. The potatoes do take a while to cook, but the nice thing about this dish is that you can just put it in the oven and forget it and then be amazed at how the flavors marry when the baking dish comes out steaming hot.

SERVES 4

STEPS

① Preheat the oven to 400°F.

② Cut the asparagus into bite-size pieces. Place in a medium-size bowl with 2 tablespoons of the olive oil, the potatoes, and salt and pepper. Toss to mix well. If it seems as if you need more oil to adequately coat all the ingredients, you can add 1 to 2 more tablespoons of oil.

③ Pour the mixture into an 8 × 8–inch baking dish and bake for 35 to 60 minutes, or until the potatoes are fork tender. (There is a large window of cook time because the size of your potato cubes can introduce some variability. Just monitor your potatoes and use them as the guide.)

④ Remove from the oven and serve.

wilted chard *with* walnut pesto *and* a balsamic reduction

There's no arguing that a traditional pesto, one made of basil, garlic, olive oil, pine nuts, and Parmesan cheese, is a timeless classic. However, we think the walnut pesto in this recipe gives the old-school classic a serious run for its money. Just be sure when making it that you add the olive and flaxseed oils *slowly*, so that you end up with the right consistency. And be warned—you might want to buy enough ingredients to make two pesto batches, because it will be hard to resist eating the pesto by itself!

SERVES 4

INGREDIENTS

2 cups (packed) flat-leaf parsley

¾ cup chopped, toasted walnuts

½ cup grated Parmesan cheese

2 tablespoons flaxseed meal

2 cloves garlic, crushed

1 cup extra virgin olive oil

2 tablespoons flaxseed oil

2 tablespoons lemon juice

1 teaspoon grated lemon zest

¾ teaspoon salt

¼ teaspoon freshly ground black pepper

½ cup balsamic vinegar

2 tablespoons grapeseed or olive oil

3 bunches rainbow chard, ribs removed, and julienned

STEPS

1 Place the parsley, walnuts, Parmesan cheese, flaxseed meal, and garlic in the bowl of a food processor or blender and process until finely chopped. With the motor running, slowly add the olive oil and flaxseed oil in a thin stream through the feed tube and process until the mixture forms a paste.

2 Remove the top and scrape down the sides of the bowl. Add the lemon juice and zest, ¾ teaspoon salt, and ¼ teaspoon pepper. Transfer the mixture to a bowl and set aside.

3 In a small saucepan over medium-high heat, reduce the balsamic vinegar by half, 6 to 7 minutes. Transfer to a small bowl and set aside.

4 In a large sauté pan, heat the grapeseed oil over medium-high heat, and when hot, add the chard and 3 tablespoons of the walnut pesto. Toss the chard with the pesto to coat and warm through, 2 to 3 minutes.

5 Transfer the chard to a serving platter and drizzle with the balsamic reduction.

6 Serve immediately.

roasted cauliflower

INGREDIENTS

1 large (about 2 pounds)
  cauliflower, cut into florets

Salt and black pepper to taste

3 tablespoons unsalted butter

1½ teaspoons minced garlic

Cauliflower is one of those vegetables that people often say they dislike without really giving it a chance. This recipe will be sure to win over some converts, although, we must admit, the butter helps! We recommend a very basic salt and pepper seasoning so you can really taste the garlic butter. However, you could always add other spices or herbs for a tasty alternative.

SERVES 4

STEPS

1 Preheat the oven to 400°F.

2 In a 13 × 9–inch baking dish, arrange the cauliflower in a single layer. Season with salt and black pepper.

3 In a small skillet, melt the butter. Add the garlic and sauté for 1 to 2 minutes.

4 Pour the butter and garlic evenly over the cauliflower and bake for 20 to 25 minutes, or until the florets begin to brown and are fork tender.

5 Remove from the oven and serve immediately.

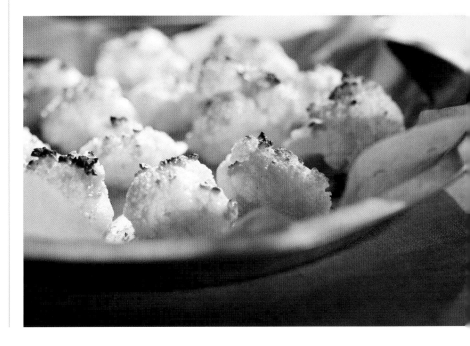

glazed carrots

INGREDIENTS

4 to 6 medium-size carrots, peeled and sliced about ¼ inch thick (about 2½ cups)

⅓ cup orange juice

¼ cup chicken or vegetable stock

2 tablespoons (packed) light brown sugar

½ teaspoon salt

Black pepper to taste

To this day, there are several dishes our mother made that we still crave, and this is one of the best. Though on busy work weeks she might serve us quick and simple meals, these carrots were one dish Mom always made from scratch. She usually made this around the holidays but it really is a welcome addition to most any meal. It goes especially well with roast meats like pork or beef, and the brown sugar and orange juice provide just enough sweetness to satisfy any palate.

SERVES 4 TO 6

STEPS

❶ Mix all the ingredients together in a medium-size skillet. Bring the liquid to a boil over medium-high heat.

❷ Reduce the heat to medium-low, cover the skillet, and simmer until the carrots are almost fork tender, about 5 minutes.

❸ Remove the cover, increase the heat to medium-high, and simmer until the liquid reduces, approximately 2 to 5 more minutes. Be sure to stir the carrots at this point so they don't burn over the higher heat.

❹ Remove from the heat, season with pepper and/or salt as desired, and serve.

sesame stir-fried rice

INGREDIENTS

1 tablespoon vegetable oil

3 tablespoons sesame oil

2 large eggs, beaten

Salt to taste

1 cup cooked brown or white rice

3 tablespoons gluten-free soy sauce or tamari

4 ounces snow peas, roughly sliced diagonally into bite-size pieces (about 1 cup)

½ teaspoon crushed red pepper flakes

Thinly sliced green onions, for garnish

This is a delicious accompaniment to so many dishes, especially our Spicy Szechuan Chicken with Cashews, Broccoli, and Green Onions (page 174). You could also serve this with a simple piece of salmon and your favorite steamed vegetables for a delicious and filling meal. We've used brown rice in this recipe to be a bit more health conscious, but feel free to use white rice instead. Get creative and experiment with different vegetables in here, too—broccoli, corn, carrots, zucchini, even nontraditional veggies like edamame and bell pepper, make for great additions. Here's to stir-fry night, everyone. Enjoy!

SERVES 4

STEPS

❶ In a medium-size saucepan or wok, heat the vegetable oil over medium heat, swirling the pan to coat the bottom evenly with the oil. Add 1 tablespoon of the sesame oil, the eggs, and a pinch of salt. Scramble the eggs until cooked through, about 3 to 4 minutes, stirring constantly.

❷ Add the cooked rice to the pan and stir well to incorporate it with the eggs.

❸ Add the remaining 2 tablespoons sesame oil and the soy sauce and stir well. Turn the heat to low.

❹ Add the snow peas, crushed red pepper flakes, and a pinch of salt. Stir well.

❺ Turn off the heat and sprinkle with the sliced green onions before giving a final stir. Serve and enjoy immediately.

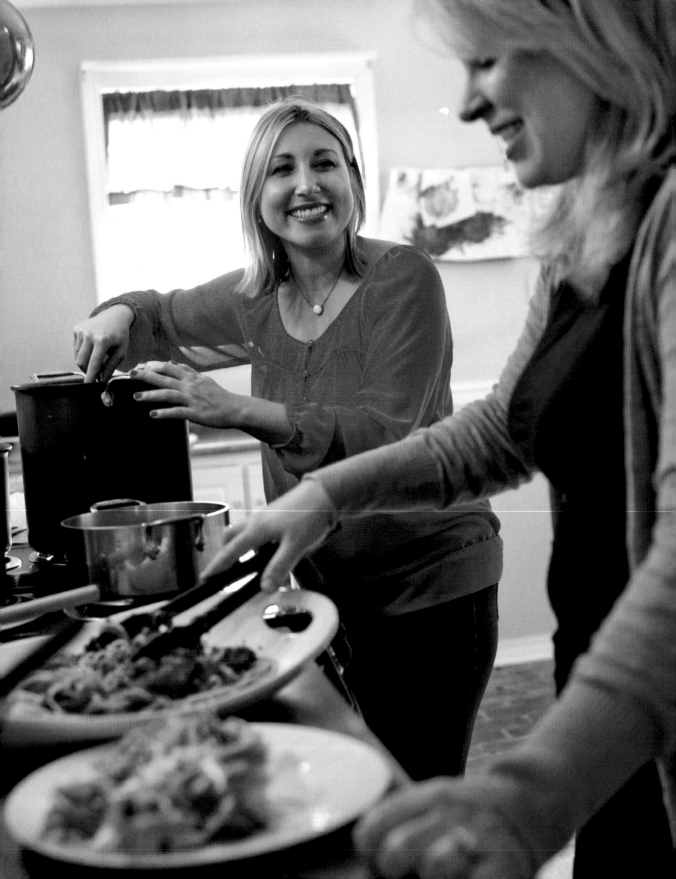

entrées

Learning to cook always needs to start somewhere, and for us entrées were the first real group of foods on which we focused. Because we each have very different food preferences, we naturally ended up with a compilation of varied entrée selections over the years. Jessie is more meat and potatoes, while Jilly is more adventurous and willing to try all different foods. So you'll have quite a range of choices here if you're looking for a new gluten-free entrée to introduce into your repertoire. Good luck!

jessie *and* jilly's jazzy jambalaya

INGREDIENTS

1 pound fresh medium-size shrimp, peeled and deveined

2 teaspoons Emeril's Original Essence Seasoning or Cajun seasoning of your choice

¼ cup olive oil

3 cloves garlic, minced

1½ pounds gluten-free andouille, sliced into bite-size rounds

1 cup chopped yellow onion

1 cup chopped celery

1 cup chopped red or yellow bell pepper

1 can (6 ounces) tomato paste

3 bay leaves

2 tablespoons fresh thyme leaves, roughly chopped

½ teaspoon dried oregano

¼ teaspoon cayenne pepper

4 cups vegetable stock or water

1 can (14 ounces) diced or chopped tomatoes

1 teaspoon celery salt

Salt and black pepper to taste

2 cups uncooked white rice

4 green onions, thinly sliced, for garnish

For anyone raised in Louisiana, this dish is pure New Orleans nostalgia in a pot. All the smells and tastes bring back wonderful memories of being children, attending Mardi Gras parades and warming up with a bowl of hot jambalaya when we got home. If andouille, or Cajun sausage, is not available to you, substitute any gluten-free smoked sausage you can find, such as Polish kielbasa. The colors of this dish, let alone the smells, will surely entice you to eat on up!

SERVES 8 TO 10

STEPS

❶ In a small bowl, combine the shrimp and Essence Seasoning. Coat all sides evenly. Set aside.

❷ In a large (10-quart) stockpot or Dutch oven, heat the oil over medium heat. Add the garlic and sausage and cook for 5 minutes to allow the sausage to brown, stirring occasionally.

❸ Add the onion, celery, bell pepper, tomato paste, bay leaves, thyme, oregano, and cayenne and stir well. Turn the heat down to low and simmer for 5 minutes.

❹ Add the stock, diced tomatoes, celery salt, and salt and black pepper to taste, stir well, and cook another 5 minutes.

❺ Add the seasoned shrimp to the pot, cover, and simmer for 3 to 4 minutes.

❻ Add the rice to the pot, stir well, and bring the mixture up to a gentle boil over medium-high heat, uncovered.

❼ Once the mixture is boiling, return the heat to low and cook 25 minutes covered, until the rice is cooked through, stirring frequently to keep the rice from sticking to the bottom of the pot.

❽ Uncover, add about ¾ of the green onions, reserving the remainder for garnish, stir well, and cook a final 5 minutes.

❾ Taste and re-season if desired. Turn off the heat and let sit covered for 10 minutes.

❿ Remove the bay leaves, if possible, before serving in bowls. Garnish with the remaining green onions.

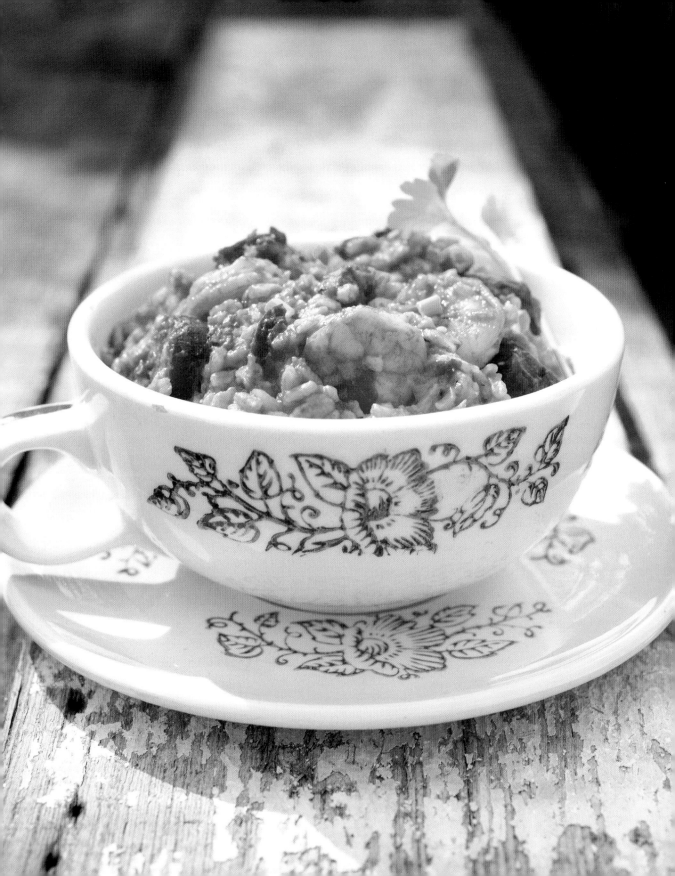

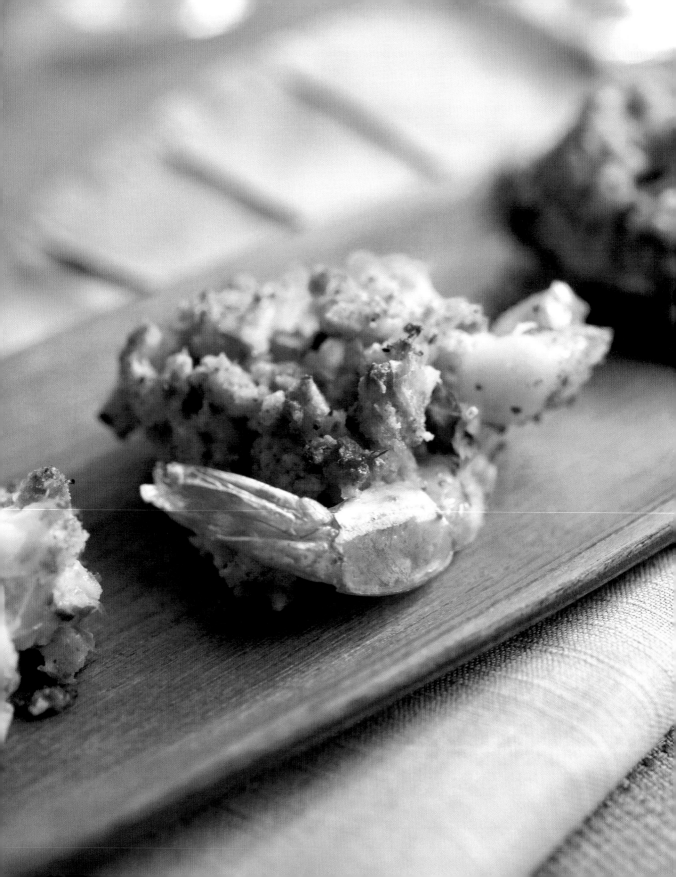

baked stuffed shrimp

INGREDIENTS

30 large shrimp, peeled and deveined

2 teaspoons olive oil

½ cup minced celery

½ cup minced yellow onion

½ cup minced green bell pepper

1 pound jumbo lump crabmeat, picked over for shells

4 teaspoons chopped fresh parsley

1 cup unseasoned gluten-free bread crumbs (see Note)

1 large egg, lightly beaten

1 cup heavy cream

1 teaspoon salt

½ teaspoon black pepper

Pinch of dried thyme

These shrimp aren't necessarily "stuffed" per se. Instead the filling is simply baked on top of the butterflied shrimp. If you really want to "stuff" them, however, you can fold one half of the shrimp over the stuffing and bake them that way. Same delicious taste, different presentation. We love this dish served with a simple rice pilaf and steamed vegetables!

SERVES 6

STEPS

1 Preheat the oven to 400°F.

2 Butterfly the shrimp by slicing them lengthwise so they can be opened flat. Do not cut all the way through; the split shrimp should remain in one piece. Lay the shrimp out in a 13 × 9–inch baking dish and set aside.

3 In a medium-size skillet, heat the olive oil over medium heat and add the celery, onion, and green pepper. Sauté until the vegetables are tender, about 5 to 7 minutes.

4 Remove from the heat and add the crabmeat and parsley. Next add the bread crumbs, egg, cream, salt, black pepper, and thyme. Mix by hand until the mixture clumps together.

5 Pile some of the mixture on top of each shrimp. Bake for 20 to 25 minutes, or until the topping becomes crispy and the shrimp are pink.

6 Remove from the oven and serve immediately.

note: *To make your own gluten-free bread crumbs, you can take 3 or 4 pieces of gluten-free bread, grind them into crumbs using a food processor, and bake them on a cookie sheet for 5 to 10 minutes at 350°F.*

pan-fried flounder
with lemon garlic butter

INGREDIENTS

2 cups buttermilk

4 flounder fillets

4 tablespoons unsalted butter, softened

1 teaspoon salt

1 teaspoon grated lemon zest

½ teaspoon finely minced green onion

½ teaspoon finely minced garlic

½ cup gluten-free all-purpose flour blend (we've used Arrowhead Mills Gluten Free All Purpose Baking Mix)

¼ teaspoon black pepper

2 tablespoons olive oil

Jessie's husband, Steven, is a true Louisianan. He loves hunting and fishing and will do either as often as possible. After one trip, he came home with tons of flounder, so Jessie concocted this recipe as a sure-fire way to make sure it all got eaten! While we like this recipe best with flounder, it also tastes great with other white, flaky fish like tilapia or haddock. It might sound odd, but soaking the fish in buttermilk will make the flesh more tender. If you have time, you might even want to soak the fillets for at least 30 minutes to really tenderize them. Yum!

SERVES 4

STEPS

① Preheat the oven to 200°F. Place an empty baking tray in the oven.

② Pour the buttermilk over the flounder fillets in a 13 × 9–inch baking dish and let them soak while you prepare the lemon garlic butter.

③ In a small bowl using a fork, cream the softened butter until it's fluffy. Add ½ teaspoon of the salt and mix well.

④ Once the salt is incorporated, add the lemon zest, green onion, and garlic, folding them into the butter until everything is evenly distributed. Cover with plastic wrap and chill.

⑤ In a second baking dish, mix together the flour blend, the remaining ½ teaspoon of salt, and pepper.

6 Dredge each fillet in the flour mixture, being sure to cover it completely. Set aside on a plate until ready to pan fry.

7 When you are ready to cook, heat 1 tablespoon of the oil in a large skillet over medium-high heat.

8 Placing 2 fillets in the skillet at a time, cook for 2 to 4 minutes per side. Be careful when flipping the fish, as it is tender and falls apart easily. It is best to use a fish flipper here, but it can be done with a regular flipper as well. Just be gentle!

9 Place the first two cooked fillets on the preheated baking tray in the oven to keep warm while you cook the remaining fillets in the remaining tablespoon of oil.

10 Place each fillet on a plate and spoon about 1 tablespoon of the butter mixture on top. The heat of the freshly cooked fish will melt the butter perfectly. Serve immediately.

prosciutto-spinach chicken roll
with lemon butter sauce

INGREDIENTS

½ cup ricotta cheese

4 teaspoons finely chopped fresh parsley

Salt and black pepper to taste

4 boneless, skinless chicken breasts, trimmed of fat

¼ pound prosciutto

1 to 2 cups spinach leaves, depending on the size of the leaves, washed and patted dry

Olive oil, as needed

3 tablespoons unsalted butter, melted (optional)

1 teaspoon grated lemon zest (optional)

2 teaspoons lemon juice (optional)

This is Jessie's twist on an old favorite, chicken Cordon Bleu. Here we replace the traditional ham and Swiss cheese with prosciutto and ricotta cheese. We also don't bread the chicken because of the way we end up assembling the roll—the prosciutto goes on the outside instead of the inside. This helps keep the chicken a bit more moist. The lemon butter sauce, while delicious and rich, is not a necessity, so don't hesitate to eliminate it if you'd prefer a lighter entrée. We really like this best when served with the lemon butter sauce and our favorite gluten-free pasta. Bon appétit!

SERVES 4

STEPS

1 Preheat the oven to 400°F.

2 Grease an 11 × 8–inch baking dish.

3 In a small bowl, stir the ricotta, parsley, salt, and pepper until thoroughly combined. Set aside.

4 Lay out the chicken breast(s) on a cutting board. You can pound one at a time or all at once, depending on the space you have available. Lay a piece of plastic wrap over the breast(s). Using a meat mallet or a rolling pin, pound each chicken breast until it is approximately the same thickness all over, between ⅛ and ¼ inch thick.

5 On a separate plastic wrap–lined cutting board or work surface, lay out 2 or 3 pieces of prosciutto per chicken breast.

6 Season the chicken with salt and pepper as desired and place each chicken breast on its allotted slices of prosciutto (see photo).

7 Using a spatula, spread the ricotta mixture evenly over the breasts, using about 2 table-spoons on each (see photo). Discard any remaining cheese once all the breasts are covered.

8 Cover the cheese layer with a single layer of spinach leaves (see photo). The bigger the leaves, the fewer you'll need.

(recipe continues)

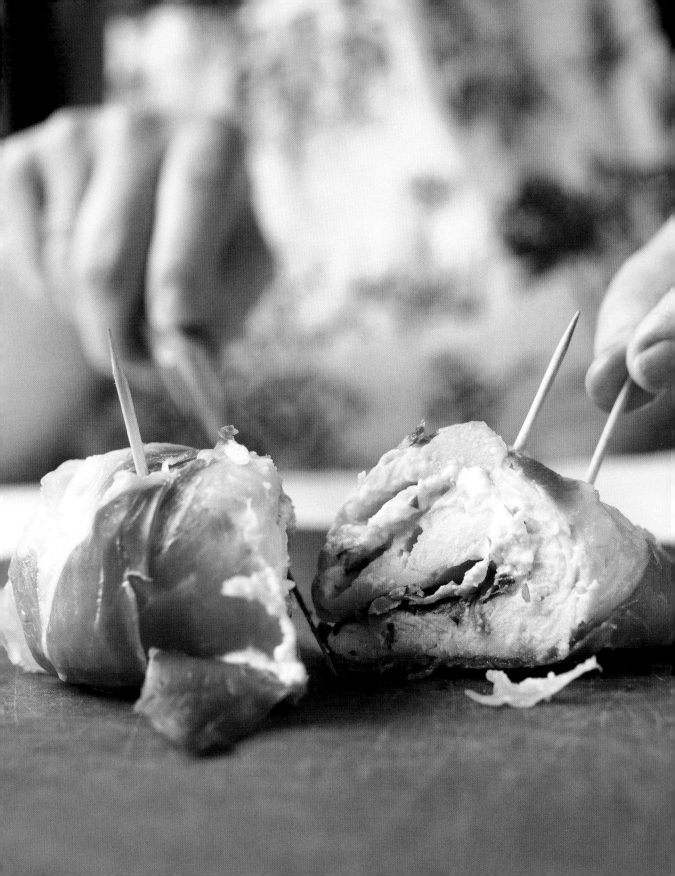

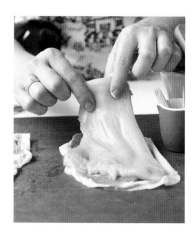 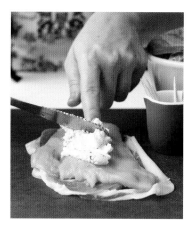 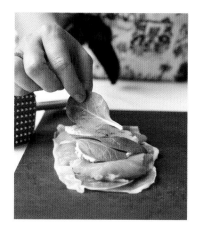

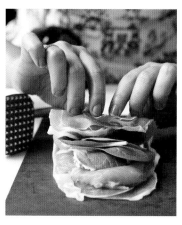 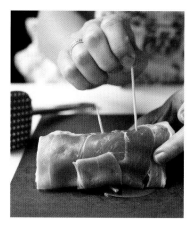

STEPS (CONT.)

9 Gently roll up each breast, being careful to keep as much of the stuffing as you can inside the roll as you go (see photo).

10 Secure with toothpicks or butcher's twine tied around the roll (see photo).

11 Drizzle enough olive oil over the breasts to coat the exterior of the rolls. Re-season with salt and pepper, if desired. Remember, you already seasoned the chicken before you rolled it up, so take that into consideration.

12 Place the rolls in the prepared baking dish and bake for 30 to 35 minutes, or until the interior is thoroughly cooked and has attained an internal temperature of 165°F. If you don't have a meat thermometer, you can always cut into one of the rolls to make sure the chicken is cooked through. (It messes up the presentation a bit, but it's better to be safe than sorry!)

13 If you choose to make the lemon butter sauce, now is the time. When the chicken has 5 to 10 minutes of baking time remaining, combine the melted butter, lemon zest, and lemon juice in a small bowl. Whisk well to blend. Set aside.

14 When the chicken rolls are ready, transfer them to serving plates. Spoon some of the lemon butter over each breast and serve immediately.

fettuccine pasta *with* prosciutto, peas, *and* cream sauce

1 pound gluten-free
   fettuccine pasta

1 tablespoon olive oil

1 tablespoon unsalted butter

¾ cup diced onion

1 tablespoon minced garlic

2 ounces prosciutto, cut into
   ¼-inch strips

¼ cup dry white wine

1½ cups heavy cream

¾ cup frozen sweet peas

¾ teaspoon salt

½ teaspoon fresh cracked
   black pepper

¾ cup grated Parmigiano-
   Reggiano cheese

¼ cup chopped fresh parsley
   leaves

As a nice alternative to a traditional tomato-based pasta sauce, this indulgent cream sauce is both easy to make and delicious to eat. The white wine really adds a nice flavor, while the prosciutto—well, honestly, prosciutto just makes everything taste better, doesn't it? Although our dad designed this recipe for fettuccine, you can certainly use any gluten-free pasta noodle you prefer. We actually like to let the pasta sit in the sauce for a few extra minutes before serving just to give the noodles a bit more time to soak up the wonderful sauce.

SERVES 6 TO 8

STEPS

❶ Cook the pasta according to package directions in boiling salted water, drain, and set aside in a large bowl until ready to use.

❷ While the pasta cooks, set a large (12-inch) sauté pan over medium-high heat and add the olive oil and the butter. Once the butter has melted, add the onion to the pan and sauté until translucent, about 3 minutes.

❸ Add the garlic to the pan and sauté for 30 seconds. Place the prosciutto in the pan and sauté for 1 minute.

❹ Deglaze the pan with the wine and cook until it is nearly evaporated, about 30 seconds.

❺ Add the cream, peas, salt, and pepper to the pan and let the cream reduce by half, 4 to 5 minutes.

❻ Pour the sauce over the pasta and sprinkle with the cheese and the parsley. Use tongs or two large forks to stir the sauce into the pasta and serve while hot.

baked halibut *with* creole tomato *and* vidalia onion vinaigrette

SERVES 4

INGREDIENTS

- 4 halibut steaks (6 to 8 ounces each), about 1 inch thick
- Olive oil to coat the fish
- Salt and black pepper
- Pinch of Emeril's Original Essence Seasoning or Cajun seasoning of your choice
- 2 large fresh, ripe tomatoes, cored and chopped (about 2 cups)
- ¼ cup extra virgin olive oil
- 3 tablespoons lemon juice
- 2 tablespoons very finely minced fresh basil
- 2 tablespoons very finely minced Vidalia onion

This is one of Jessie's favorite summer dishes and a big hit with our little brother and sister, too! Fresh and ripe Creole tomatoes provide a great balance to the sweet Vidalia onions. If you can't get Creole tomatoes or Vidalia onions, you can work with regular tomatoes and a different kind of onion, but don't forget the seasoning to give it an extra kick. We hope you find this dish as refreshing as we do!

STEPS

1 Preheat the oven to 400°F.

2 Coat the halibut steaks with olive oil and season each with a dash of salt, pepper, and Essence Seasoning.

3 Place the steaks side by side in a 13 × 9–inch baking dish and bake for 15 to 25 minutes, or until the fish flakes when pressed with a fork.

4 While the halibut is cooking, mix the tomatoes with ½ teaspoon salt and ¼ teaspoon pepper in a medium-size bowl. Set aside.

5 In another medium-size bowl, whisk the extra virgin olive oil with the lemon juice. Add the basil and onion and whisk again until incorporated. Stir the tomato mixture into the oil mixture.

6 Remove the halibut from the oven and place one steak on each of 4 serving plates. Spoon about ½ cup of the tomato mixture over each steak and serve.

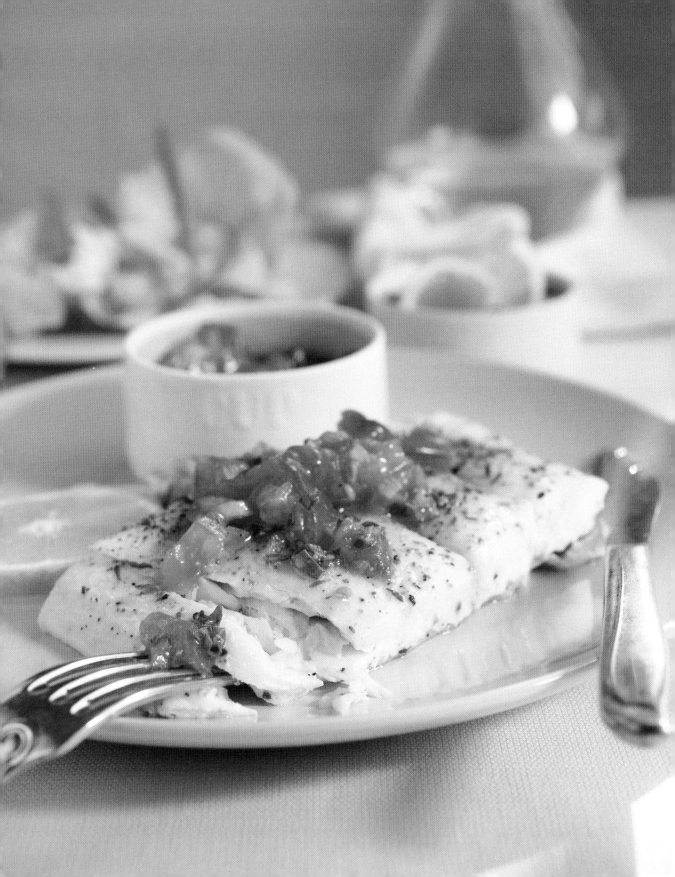

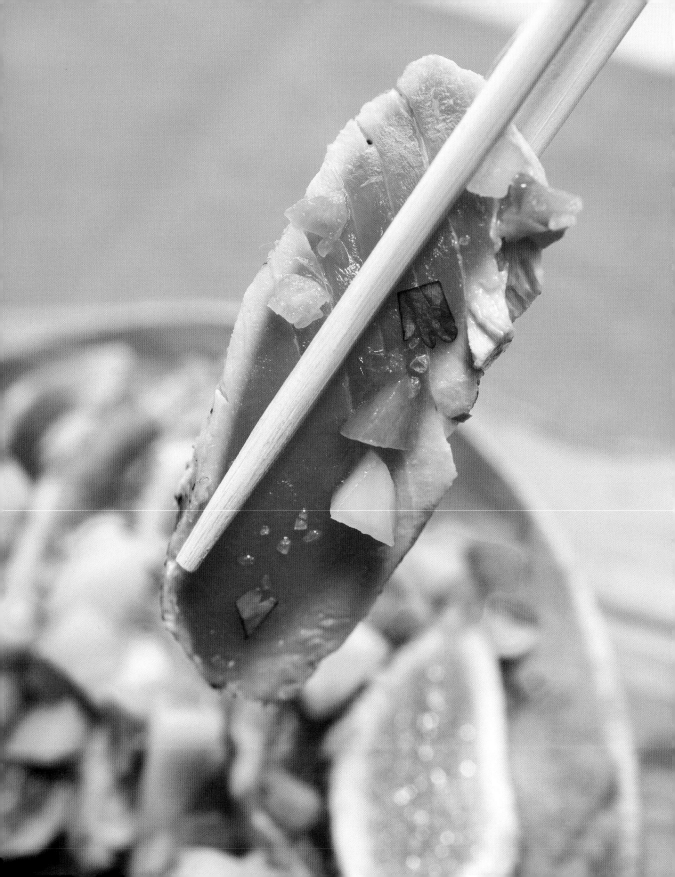

grilled tuna *with* mango salsa

INGREDIENTS

¼ cup olive oil

3 tablespoons lemon juice

¼ teaspoon salt

¼ teaspoon black pepper

4 tuna steaks (4 to 6 ounces each), about 1 inch thick

1 cup roughly chopped fresh mango

2 tablespoons finely diced yellow bell pepper

2 tablespoons finely diced red bell pepper

2 tablespoons finely diced red onion

1 teaspoon chopped fresh cilantro

Our dad taught Jessie to make a version of this dish when she was first learning how to cook fish. There's something about the wonderful sweetness of the mango salsa paired with the fresh, peppery tuna that simply hits the spot. Like a few of our other recipes, this one works great on an indoor grill as well as an outdoor one. If grilling indoors on a two-sided grill, the cooking time should be reduced by as much as half, since no turning is required.

SERVES 4

STEPS

❶ In a large Ziploc bag or a baking dish, combine the olive oil, lemon juice, salt, and black pepper. Add the tuna steaks and marinate for no more than 30 minutes before grilling. (Any longer and you run the risk that the lemon juice will gradually start to cook the fish, giving it a tough consistency.)

❷ While the tuna is marinating, make a salsa by combining the remaining ingredients— the mango, yellow and red bell peppers, red onion, and cilantro—in a small bowl. Toss thoroughly to mix. Refrigerate.

❸ When you are ready to cook the tuna, grill it for 3 to 5 minutes on each side. It should be light brownish on the outside but remain pink on the inside.

❹ Spoon some of the salsa on top of each steak and serve.

red beans *and* rice

INGREDIENTS

2 tablespoons olive oil

2 cups diced yellow onion

1 cup diced celery

1 cup diced green bell pepper

1 tablespoon minced garlic

1 pound dried red beans,
  soaked in water for
  24 hours, then drained

1 ham hock (about ½ pound)

1 pound cooked ham, diced

1 teaspoon cayenne pepper

1 teaspoon black pepper

1 bay leaf

8 cups chicken stock or water

2 teaspoons salt, or as needed
  (see Note)

2 cups cooked white rice

Sliced green onion, for garnish
  (optional)

In New Orleans, following a deep-rooted Creole tradition, many restaurants and families still serve red beans and rice on Monday. Don't worry, though! It can still be found on the other six days of the week. The story goes as follows: Years ago, when pork was the traditional Sunday dinner meat and Monday was clothes-washing day, the local women needed a meal that could both use the leftover pork from the previous night and not require much attending, since they needed to be washing clothes and not hovering over the stove. Thus, red beans and rice became the dish of choice to make on Mondays. In staying true to tradition, this recipe uses chunks of ham and a ham hock to impart some nice, meaty flavor. We recommend soaking your beans for a day before cooking them—it will help them cook faster. Enjoy!

SERVES 4 TO 6

STEPS

1 In a medium-size (6-quart) stockpot over medium heat, heat the olive oil. Add the onion, celery, green pepper, and garlic and sauté until they begin to soften, about 5 minutes.

2 Add the beans, ham hock, diced ham, cayenne, black pepper, and bay leaf along with the stock or water. Simmer uncovered for 1½ to 2 hours, or until the liquid is thick and the beans have split open. If the 8 cups of liquid are absorbed before the beans are tender, you can add 1 or 2 more cups to help the beans finish cooking.

3 Add salt as necessary, adjust the seasoning, and remove the bay leaf. Some people like to break up the meat on the ham hock and incorporate it into the beans. If you'd like to do that, now would be the time. Once the meat is removed, discard what's left of the ham hock. Serve the beans over the cooked rice, garnished, if desired, with sliced green onion.

note: *The ham or ham hock you use might already have some salt in it. We recommend waiting until the beans are almost fully cooked before adding salt. That way, you can taste the effect of the salted ham and you don't end up with too much salt!'*

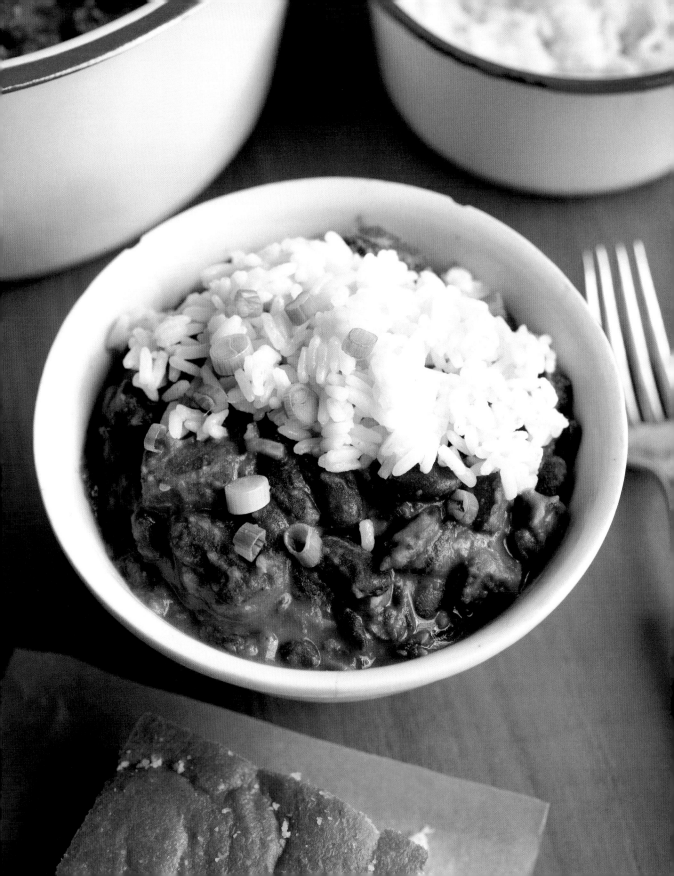

baked stuffed peppers

INGREDIENTS

2 cups water

1 tablespoon lightly salted butter

1 cup white or brown quick-cooking rice (10-minute variety)

Salt

2 to 3 tablespoons olive oil

1 small yellow onion, chopped

2 medium-size stalks celery, trimmed, halved lengthwise, and chopped

1 green bell pepper, cored, seeded, and chopped

½ cup finely chopped cremini, or baby bella, mushrooms

1 clove garlic, minced

Black pepper to taste

1 pound lean ground turkey

2 teaspoons Emeril's Original Essence Seasoning or Cajun seasoning of your choice

1½ teaspoons fresh thyme leaves, roughly chopped

2 cans (14 ounces each) diced or chopped tomatoes

8 to 10 medium-size bell peppers, any color preferred like red, yellow or green, left whole but cored, seeded, and ribs removed

Freshly grated Parmesan cheese (optional)

These peppers are packed with flavor. This is a quick and easy dish to put together, and it's so filling there may even be leftovers so you can take tomorrow night off! Use any combination of vegetables you like for the stuffing mixture, and feel free to prepare it a day in advance and bake as needed. You can experiment with the colors of bell peppers and the type of ground meat, for different flavor combinations. Perhaps try ground beef or even lamb instead, for an exotic twist. Jessie loves these peppers served alongside a big, crisp salad. Jilly prefers hers with loads of nutty grated Parmesan cheese on top. However you serve it up, this will be one nutritious and delicious dinner that everyone in your family will enjoy.

MAKES 8 TO 10 PEPPERS

STEPS

❶ Preheat the oven to 375°F.

❷ In a medium-size saucepan, combine the water and butter and bring to a boil over medium-high heat.

❸ Add the rice and cook according to package directions, seasoning with salt, if desired. Set aside.

❹ In a large sauté pan with deep sides, heat the olive oil over medium heat. Add the onion, celery, chopped bell pepper, mushrooms, and garlic to the pan, season with salt and pepper, and sauté until the vegetables are slightly softened, about 6 to 8 minutes.

❺ Add the ground turkey, Essence Seasoning, and thyme to the pan and sauté until the meat

is fully cooked, making sure to crumble it with a wooden spoon as it cooks.

❻ Once the meat is fully cooked through, add the tomatoes to the pan and stir well.

❼ Add the cooked rice to the meat mixture and stir until thoroughly combined. Taste and re-season if needed. Turn off the heat.

❽ Arrange the prepared peppers in a baking dish with deep sides. You want the peppers to stand upright in the dish without falling.

❾ Spoon some meat-and-rice mixture into each pepper, packing it down as you go and distributing the mixture evenly among the peppers. Once filled,

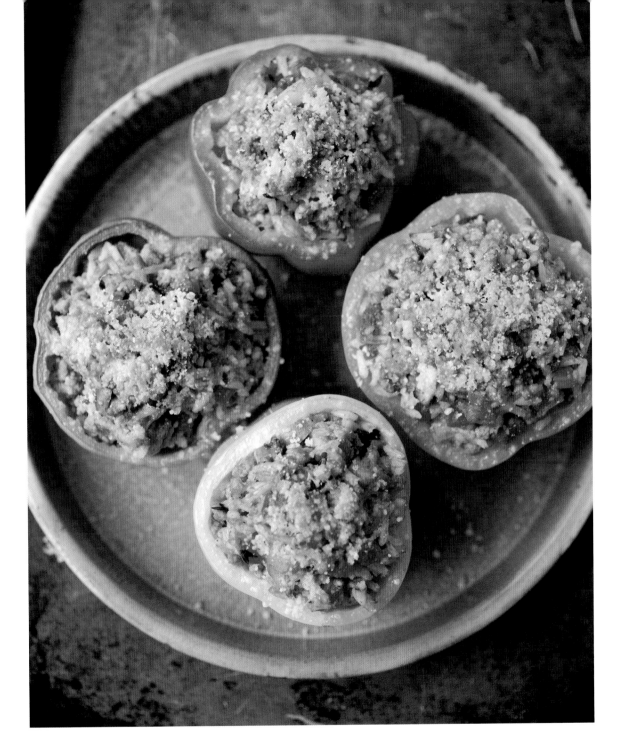

sprinkle a generous amount of grated Parmesan on each pepper, if you'd like.

10 Bake for 25 to 30 minutes, or until filling is golden brown on top and the peppers are a bit soft.

11 Remove from the oven and serve.

cornbread *and* andouille stuffed pork chops

INGREDIENTS

cornbread

¾ cup yellow cornmeal

¾ cup gluten-free all-purpose flour blend (we've used Arrowhead Mills Gluten Free All Purpose Baking Mix)

1 tablespoon gluten-free baking powder

¼ teaspoon salt, or to taste

¼ teaspoon pepper, or to taste

¾ cup buttermilk (see Note)

1 large egg

¼ cup vegetable oil

dressing

2 tablespoons olive oil

¾ pound gluten-free andouille sausage, chopped into bite-size pieces

¾ cup diced yellow onion

¾ cup thinly sliced green onions (about 4 green onions)

⅓ cup diced celery

⅓ cup diced green bell pepper

3 tablespoons minced garlic

Enough cornbread for 4 cups, crumbled

1 to 2 cups chicken stock

2 teaspoons Emeril's Original Essence Seasoning or Cajun seasoning of your choice

---

Yum! It's hard to not like stuffed pork chops—especially when they come chock full of our favorite cornbread-andouille dressing (or what some people call stuffing: any sort of bread-based mixture of goodness). Technically, any dressing would work for this recipe, but there's something about the down-home flavors of savory cornbread and spicy Cajun andouille sausage that makes us melt. The dressing is also good on its own, as a side to whatever your favorite meat-and-veggie combo is. When stuffing any meat, be sure to ask your butcher to cut the stuffing pockets into the pork for you. Butchers are usually experts at this, and it makes the recipe that much easier!

SERVES 6

STEPS

cornbread

1 Preheat the oven to 425°F.

2 Grease an 8 × 8–inch baking pan.

3 In a large bowl, combine the cornmeal, flour blend, baking powder, salt, and pepper.

4 Add the buttermilk, egg, and oil. Beat with a fork until fairly smooth and all the ingredients are incorporated, about 1 minute.

5 Pour the batter into the prepared baking pan and bake 20 to 25 minutes, or until a toothpick inserted in the center comes out clean. Remove from the oven and let cool.

dressing

1 Preheat the oven to 375°F.

2 Grease an 8 × 8–inch baking pan.

3 In a large skillet over medium heat, heat the olive oil. Add the sausage and onion and sauté until the onion is softened, about 5 to 7 minutes.

4 Add the green onions, celery, bell pepper, and garlic and cook until the bell pepper is softened, about 5 to 7 more minutes. Stir often to keep the ingredients from burning.

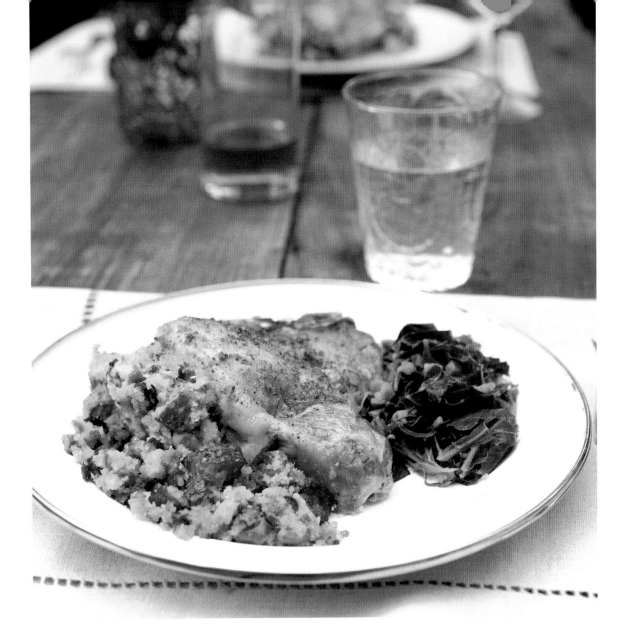

5 While the vegetables and sausage are cooking, crumble enough of the cooled cornbread to make 4 cups into a large bowl.

6 Stir the sautéed vegetables, chicken stock, and Essence Seasoning into the cornbread to thoroughly mix. You can use as much or as little chicken stock as you want to get your dressing the consistency you prefer. We usually like about 1½ cups of stock in ours.

7 Transfer the cornbread mixture to the prepared baking pan and bake until the top is crispy, about 30 minutes. Remove from the oven and let cool.

(recipe continues)

pork chops

6 pork chops, each 1 to
1½ inches thick

1 to 2 tablespoons olive oil, or
enough to coat each side of
each pork chop

1 tablespoon salt

1 tablespoon black pepper

1 tablespoon Emeril's Original
Essence Seasoning or Cajun
seasoning of your choice

note: *If you don't have*
buttermilk, place 1 tablespoon
of white vinegar in a
measuring cup. Add enough
whole milk to the measuring
cup to bring the total amount
of liquid to 1 cup. Let sit for
10 minutes. Stir and use this
instead of buttermilk.

pork chops

❶ Once the cornbread dressing has cooled to a manageable temperature, preheat the oven to 350°F.

❷ Grease a baking tray.

❸ Starting with the pork chops lying on a cutting board, slice a 2- to 3-inch horizontal cut into the nonbone side of each chop. Slice about two-thirds of the way through the chop, stopping before your knife hits the bone. The slice should create a pocket within the chop. (Skip this step if your butcher made the pockets for you.)

❹ Coat both sides of each pork chop with olive oil. Season with salt, pepper, and Essence Seasoning.

❺ Using a spoon or your hands, stuff the pocket with as much of the cornbread andouille dressing as will fit, usually anywhere from ½ to ¾ cup of dressing, depending on the pork chop and pocket size.

❻ Place the stuffed pork chops on the prepared baking tray and bake for 35 to 40 minutes, or until the pork's internal temperature reaches 145°F. The time will vary depending on the chops' thickness.

maple-glazed pork loin *with* rosemary, thyme, *and* green onions

INGREDIENTS

1 boneless pork loin (between 2 and 2½ pounds)

½ teaspoon salt

¼ teaspoon black pepper

1 cup chopped green onions (about 5 green onions)

⅔ cup maple syrup

1 tablespoon fresh rosemary leaves, minced

2 teaspoons dried thyme

Our stepfather, Ed, was a born-and-raised Vermonter and, understandably, a huge maple syrup fan. He'd put it on ground beef, chicken, even popcorn! For this recipe, we added maple syrup to a pork loin glaze and produced some delicious pork. To maximize your sweet, syrupy flavors, remember to baste the loin with the glaze every so often or roll the loin in the glaze, using tongs, so it reaches every part of the pork.

SERVES 4 TO 6

STEPS

1 Preheat the oven to 375°F.

2 Remove, as best you can, the pork "silver," the shiny film of muscle or tendon that is sometimes on the edge of the pork loin. Sprinkle the salt and pepper evenly over the pork and place it in a 13 × 9–inch baking dish.

3 In a small bowl, mix the green onions, maple syrup, rosemary, and thyme. Pour over the pork loin and place the baking dish in the oven.

4 Cook for 40 to 50 minutes, or until the internal temperature reaches 145°F. Be sure to baste or turn the roast every 15 minutes.

5 When the pork is thoroughly cooked, remove the baking dish from the oven and let the pork sit for 5 to 10 minutes so the glaze can thicken slightly.

6 Transfer the pork to a cutting board and cut into ¼- to ½-inch slices. Arrange the slices on plates or a serving dish.

7 Pour some of the remaining glaze over the slices and serve.

smothered pork chops

INGREDIENTS

4 thin-cut pork chops

Emeril's Original Essence Seasoning or Cajun seasoning of your choice, to taste

½ teaspoon salt, plus more to taste

¼ teaspoon black pepper, plus more to taste

2 tablespoons olive oil, plus more as needed for the roux

2 tablespoons gluten-free all-purpose flour blend (we've used Arrowhead Mills Gluten Free All Purpose Baking Mix)

1 large yellow onion, thinly sliced (about 1½ cups)

3 to 3½ cups chicken stock

1 bay leaf

1 tablespoon cornstarch mixed with 1 tablespoon water (optional)

1 pound gluten-free smoked sausage, sliced

1 medium-size potato, peeled and diced (1⅓ to 1½ cups)

Our dad taught us a version of this delicious pork chop recipe a few years ago and we've been hooked ever since. As we are sure you will find, this relatively easy dish quickly becomes a favorite treatment for pork. It is delicious and quite filling—and you can even up your carbohydrate load by serving the whole thing over steamed rice. You can use a bone-in chop or a boneless one to suit your preference. Also, if you don't have Emeril's Original Essence Seasoning, you can substitute a similar Cajun spice as desired.

SERVES 4

STEPS

❶ Season both sides of each pork chop with several sprinkles of Essence Seasoning, salt, and pepper.

❷ In a large skillet over medium-high heat, heat the olive oil and sear the chops for 2 to 4 minutes on each side, or until they begin to brown.

❸ Remove the chops from the skillet and set aside. Lower the heat to medium and add more olive oil until you estimate that there is again about 2 tablespoons of oil in the pan.

❹ Add the flour blend and cook for another 2 to 4 minutes, stirring constantly so the roux doesn't burn. The mixture should turn the color of light peanut butter.

❺ Add the onion, ½ teaspoon salt, and ¼ teaspoon pepper and cook another 5 minutes, or until the onions have softened and are coated with the roux.

❻ Stir in 2⅔ cups of the chicken stock until the roux mixture has blended smoothly into the stock.

❼ Return the pork chops to the skillet, along with the bay leaf, and cover. Simmer on low heat for 30 to 45 minutes, stirring the roux mixture occasionally. If the gravy becomes too thick, add enough of the remaining chicken stock to thin it out. If the gravy is too thin, incorporate the cornstarch and water mixture to thicken it up.

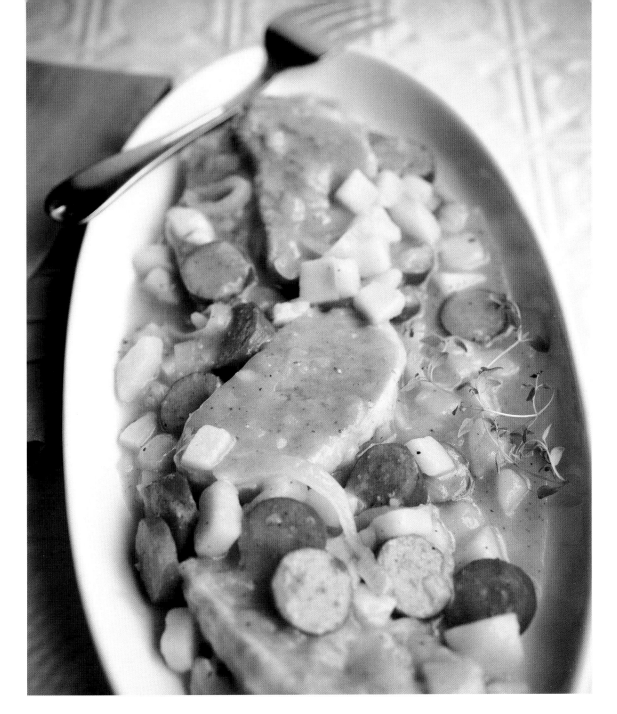

❽ After the chops have simmered for 30 to 45 minutes, add the sliced sausage and diced potatoes. Re-season the mixture, re-cover, and simmer for an additional 10 to 15 minutes, or until the potatoes are tender.

❾ Remove from the heat and discard the bay leaf. Serve each chop with a heaping pile of sausage and potatoes along with a healthy spoonful of gravy.

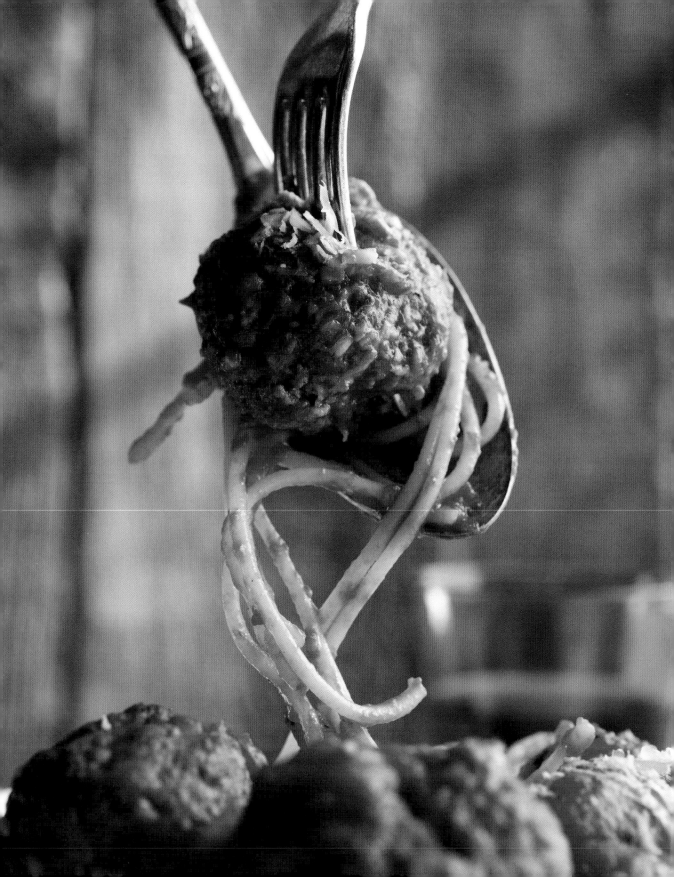

spaghetti *with* meatballs

INGREDIENTS

meatballs

1 medium-size white onion, quartered

½ cup gluten-free bread crumbs or 2 slices gluten-free bread, toasted

¼ cup buttermilk

1½ pounds lean ground beef

1 large egg

½ cup freshly grated Parmesan cheese

1 teaspoon salt

1 teaspoon black pepper

1 tablespoon chopped fresh parsley

1 tablespoon minced garlic

sauce

2 tablespoons olive oil

2 cups chopped yellow onion (about 2 medium-size onions)

2 teaspoons minced garlic

2 cans (15 ounces) plain tomato sauce

1 can (15 ounces) diced tomatoes

Water (one 15-ounce can's worth)

2 teaspoons finely chopped fresh basil

2 teaspoons dried oregano

2 bay leaves

¼ teaspoon black pepper, or more to taste

Salt to taste

This red sauce was one of the first dishes our father taught us to make. Over the years we've tweaked it a bit until we got it just where we like it! The gluten-free meatballs come out terrifically, too. For the meatballs, the gluten-free bread crumbs can be store-bought if you can find them, but we usually make our own.

Serve the meatballs and sauce over gluten-free spaghetti or another gluten-free pasta of your choice, enough to feed 6.

SERVES 6 (MAKES ABOUT TWENTY-FOUR 1- TO 1½-INCH MEATBALLS)

STEPS

meatballs

1 Preheat the oven to 375°F.

2 Process the onion in a food processor until pureed; you should have about ¾ cup. If using toasted gluten-free bread instead of bread crumbs, process the bread and the buttermilk along with the onion.

3 In a large mixing bowl, combine all the ingredients. Mix by hand until the mixture becomes one uniformly textured mass.

4 Scoop the mixture out and roll into 1- to 1½-inch balls. Place on a greased baking tray and bake for 15 to 20 minutes, or until the meatballs have firmed up to the point where they maintain their shape (see Note).

5 Remove the meatballs from the oven and cool until it is time to add them to the sauce.

sauce

1 While the meatballs are cooking, heat the olive oil in a medium-size (6-quart) stockpot. Add the onion and garlic and sauté for 3 to 5 minutes, or until the onion begins to soften.

2 Add all the other ingredients and stir to mix. Cook over medium-low heat for 30 minutes, and then add the meatballs. Cook for another 15 minutes, or until the sauce has thickened to your desired consistency.

3 Remove the bay leaf before spooning over cooked pasta of your choice. Enjoy!

note: For a crispier meatball, cook the meatballs on the stovetop, in olive oil in a large skillet over medium-high heat, until the outsides are browned and crispy.

prosciutto *and* herb rigatoni

1 large bunch asparagus

1 pound gluten-free rigatoni or gluten-free pasta of your choice

2 cups chicken stock

¼ cup cornstarch

¼ cup olive oil

1 teaspoon finely chopped garlic

1 cup chopped onion

6 ounces prosciutto, diced

4 medium-size sun-dried tomatoes in olive oil, chopped

2 tablespoons sliced fresh basil leaves

2 tablespoons coarsely chopped fresh parsley

1 tablespoon chopped fresh dill

Salt and black pepper to taste

Freshly grated Parmesan cheese to taste

This delicious pasta dish seems so decadent, but since the sauce is made with cornstarch rather than cream or a roux, it's really quite healthy. While we prefer gluten-free rigatoni as the pasta here, the entrée can be made with whichever gluten-free noodle is your favorite. The herbed sauce comes out pretty thick, so if you'd prefer more of a broth than a sauce, add some extra chicken stock.

SERVES 4

STEPS

1 Cut off and discard the tough ends of the asparagus and slice the remainder into 1-inch pieces. Blanch in a saucepan of boiling water for 30 seconds. Drain and run under cold water for a minute or so, and then set aside to cool further.

2 While the asparagus is cooling, cook the pasta in a large (8-quart) stockpot of boiling water until tender but still al dente or somewhat firm, approximately 10 minutes. Drain and set aside.

3 Bring 1 cup of the chicken stock to a boil in a medium-size saucepan. While the stock is coming to a boil, whisk the remaining stock into the cornstarch in a small bowl. Whisk the cornstarch mixture into the boiling stock. Stirring constantly, cook until thickened. The mixture will thicken quite quickly, so be sure to keep whisking! Once it has thickened, remove from the heat and set aside.

4 In a large heavy saucepan over medium-high heat, heat the olive oil. Add the garlic and onion and sauté until the onion begins to soften, about 3 to 5 minutes.

5 Add the prosciutto, tomatoes, basil, parsley, dill, asparagus, salt, and pepper. Sauté for another 2 to 4 minutes.

6 Add the thickened chicken stock to the saucepan and bring to a simmer. Stir in the pasta, making sure it is evenly coated with the sauce. Cook briefly to reheat the pasta, 2 minutes or so. If you get to this point and you think the sauce is too thick for your liking, feel free to add some more chicken stock to get it to your desired consistency.

7 Transfer the pasta to a serving bowl, sprinkle with grated Parmesan, and serve immediately.

polenta-baked chicken tenders

INGREDIENTS

1 pound boneless, skinless chicken tender pieces

½ cup buttermilk

¾ cup polenta, or coarsely ground cornmeal

1 tablespoon Emeril's Original Essence Seasoning or Cajun seasoning of your choice

Salt and black pepper to taste

Kids and grown-ups alike will love these tasty lil' tenders. Who doesn't love a crispy and succulent chicken tender? The buttermilk in this recipe makes the chicken stay moist. This is a great gluten-free take on an American classic, and much healthier, since we bake the tenders as opposed to frying them. The polenta breading mixture is excellent on your favorite white-fleshed fish as well. Jessie likes to add a bit of honey to the mixture for—yes—honey-sweet tenders, which her son Jude can't seem to get enough of. The possibilities are endless! For a complete Southern meal, serve with our Sour Cream and Chive Mash (page 114) and our Green Beans with Bacon and Onions (page 110). Dunk these little babies in anything your heart desires, or try them wrapped up in corn tortillas, with some salsa or guacamole, for a Latin twist.

SERVES 4

STEPS

❶ In a medium-size bowl, combine the chicken pieces and the buttermilk and toss well to make sure the chicken is thoroughly coated. Cover, place in the refrigerator, and marinate for 15 to 30 minutes.

❷ Meanwhile, preheat the oven to 375°F.

❸ Lightly grease a baking tray.

❹ In another medium-size bowl, combine the polenta, Essence Seasoning, and salt and pepper to taste. Stir well.

❺ Remove the chicken from the refrigerator. Dredge each tender in the polenta mixture, making sure it's well coated on all sides, and place on the prepared baking tray. Discard any remaining polenta mixture.

❻ Bake for 25 to 30 minutes, depending on the size of the tenders, until cooked through, flipping once halfway through the cooking time to allow both sides of the chicken to crisp.

❼ Serve with your favorite dipping sauce.

spaghetti bolognese

INGREDIENTS

1 tablespoon olive oil

4 ounces bacon or pancetta, diced

1½ cups chopped yellow onion

¾ cup diced carrot

¾ cup diced celery

1 tablespoon minced garlic

1 teaspoon salt

½ teaspoon ground black pepper

2 bay leaves

½ teaspoon dried thyme

¼ teaspoon dried oregano

½ teaspoon ground cinnamon

½ teaspoon ground nutmeg

1 pound ground beef or ground veal

½ pound gluten-free pork sausage, removed from the casings, or ground pork

2 tablespoons tomato paste

1 cup red wine

2 cans (14½ ounces each) crushed tomatoes and their juice

1 can (14½ ounces) tomato sauce

1 cup beef or chicken stock or broth

2 teaspoons sugar

¼ cup heavy cream

2 tablespoons unsalted butter

3 tablespoons chopped fresh parsley leaves

1 pound gluten-free spaghetti

1 cup freshly grated Parmesan cheese

Recipe courtesy Emeril Lagasse, copyright MSLO Inc., all rights reserved.

Years ago, when we were still in high school in Massachusetts and our dad first began spending time in New York City for work, we'd sometimes get to go into the city to visit him. Whenever we did so, he'd treat us to a wonderful dinner at a small Italian restaurant near his hotel. They had the most mouth-watering spaghetti Bolognese, creamy yet tangy, with just enough meaty chunkiness. It was just delicious! This version of Bolognese is as close as we've been able to get to those yummy flavors of our memory. We hope you enjoy it as much as we do.

SERVES 6 TO 8

STEPS

❶ In a large pot, heat the oil over medium-high heat. Add the bacon and cook, stirring, until browned and the fat is rendered, 4 to 5 minutes.

❷ Add the onion, carrot, and celery and cook, stirring, until soft, 4 to 5 minutes.

❸ Add the garlic, salt, pepper, bay leaves, thyme, oregano, cinnamon, and nutmeg and cook, stirring, for 30 seconds.

❹ Add the beef and sausages, and cook, stirring, until no longer pink, about 5 minutes.

❺ Add the tomato paste and cook, stirring, for 1 to 2 minutes.

❻ Add the wine and cook, stirring, to deglaze the pan and remove any browned bits sticking to the bottom of the pan, and until half of the liquid is evaporated, about 2 minutes.

❼ Add the tomatoes and their juice, the tomato sauce, beef broth, and sugar and bring to a boil. Reduce the heat to medium low and simmer, stirring occasionally to keep the sauce from sticking to the bottom of the pan, until the sauce is thickened and flavorful, about 1½ hours.

❽ Add the cream, butter, and parsley, stir well, and simmer for 2 minutes.

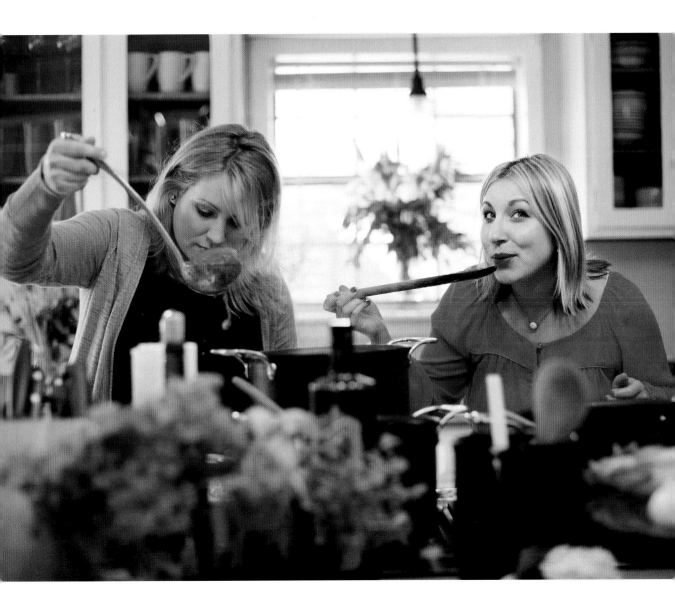

9 Discard the bay leaves and adjust the seasoning to taste. Remove from the heat and cover to keep warm until ready to serve.

10 Meanwhile, bring a large pot of salted water to a boil. Add the pasta and return the water to a low boil. Cook, stirring occasionally, to prevent the noodles from sticking, until al dente, 8 to 10 minutes. Drain in a colander.

11 Add the pasta to the sauce, tossing to coat. Add 1/2 cup of the cheese and toss to blend.

Divide among pasta bowls and serve with the remaining cheese passed tableside. (Alternatively, toss only the desired portion of pasta with a bit of the sauce at a time in a serving bowl, reserving the remainder for another meal.)

lemon *and* asparagus risotto

INGREDIENTS

1 pound fresh asparagus, thoroughly washed and patted dry

4 cups chicken or vegetable stock

Salt to taste

3 tablespoons olive oil

2 cloves garlic, minced

2 shallots or 1 small yellow onion, finely diced

2 tablespoons lightly salted butter

1 cup Arborio or Carnaroli risotto rice

Finely grated zest and juice of 1 lemon

¼ cup freshly grated Parmesan cheese

Black pepper to taste

Extra virgin olive oil for serving (optional)

We simply adore this naturally gluten-free dish, which to us just screams, "Spring has sprung." This is a delicious springtime meal to make when asparagus is in its peak season, so try going to your local farmer's market for the freshest bunch you can find. This may seem like a lot of work for risotto. Trust us that the end result is well worth the effort. The gorgeous asparagus flavor is layered throughout the dish. Since we use the stems to make our stock, nothing is wasted here. As for the risotto rice, there are three different types of risotto rice to choose from: Vialone, which is the smallest grain of the three; Carnaroli, which is sized somewhere in the middle; and Arborio, which is the most commonly used and the largest of the three. We suggest using either Arborio or Carnaroli for this particular recipe.

SERVES 4

STEPS

❶ Trim the hard ends of the asparagus and discard. Using a vegetable peeler, gently peel off the tough skin on the lower part of the stem. (Start about halfway down from the tip.)

❷ Discard the peelings and cut each stem in half across the middle.

❸ Roughly chop the lower half of the stems you've just cut. Set aside. We'll use this to make our stock.

❹ Cut the tips off the upper asparagus halves and slice the stems into small, pea-size pieces. Set aside.

❺ Divide the chicken stock evenly between 2 medium-size saucepans and bring one to a boil over high heat. Bring the second to a boil over low heat.

❻ Once the first pot is boiling, add the chopped stalks and a pinch of salt to it. Return to a boil.

❼ Cover, turn the heat to low, and simmer until the stems are tender, about 10 minutes, depending on thickness and size.

❽ Meanwhile, keep the other pan of stock simmering gently on low heat until needed.

❾ In a large sauté pan with deep sides, heat the olive oil with the garlic over low heat.

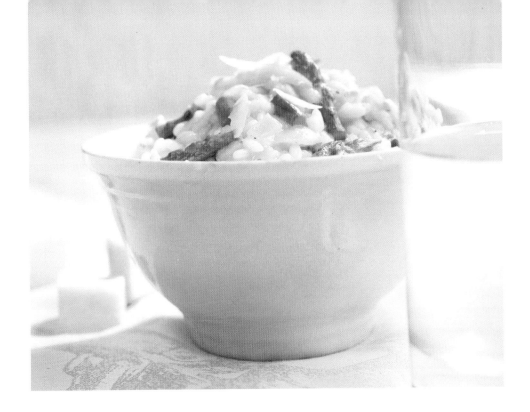

⑩ Add the shallots and sauté gently until soft, about 4 minutes.

⑪ Add the reserved asparagus tips and pea-size stem pieces from step 4 above, the butter, and a pinch of salt and cook another 3 minutes.

⑫ Add the rice to the pan, stirring well to make sure it is well coated.

⑬ Sauté for 2 minutes before stirring in 2 to 3 ladlefuls of the plain stock that has been simmering.

⑭ Stir the risotto mixture constantly until the stock is absorbed. Then, add the remaining stock 2 to 3 ladlefuls at a time and stir until the rice has absorbed all the liquid. This should take 8 to 10 minutes.

⑮ Meanwhile, pour the chopped asparagus stems and stock from the other saucepan into a blender. Place a kitchen towel over the lid and hold down firmly while blending, as hot liquids expand and tend to want to shoot out the top. *Carefully* blend until smooth.

⑯ Stir the pureed mixture, along with the lemon juice and zest, into the risotto pan, mix well, and increase the heat to medium low. Cook another 20 minutes uncovered, stirring occasionally. You want all the stock and puree mixture to be absorbed. The rice should be cooked but maintain a slight, al dente bite. It should *not* be mushy.

⑰ After the 20 minutes, stir in the grated Parmesan with a generous bit of pepper and more salt, if desired.

⑱ Turn off the heat and serve immediately, drizzled with a bit of extra virgin olive oil, if desired.

chicken pot pie
with lyonnaise potato crust

INGREDIENTS

¾ pound boneless, skinless chicken breasts, diced into bite-size chunks

1½ tablespoons Emeril's Original Essence Seasoning or Cajun seasoning of your choice

1½ tablespoons olive oil

6 tablespoons unsalted butter

1 cup chopped yellow onion

½ cup chopped celery

2 cloves garlic, minced

Salt and black pepper to taste

¼ cup plus 2 tablespoons gluten-free all-purpose flour blend (we've used Arrowhead Mills Gluten Free All Purpose Baking Mix)

1½ cups chicken or vegetable stock

1½ cups dry white wine or additional stock

1 cup half-and-half

1 cup diced carrot, blanched in boiling water 4 minutes and drained

1 cup frozen peas

1½ tablespoons fresh thyme leaves, preferably lemon thyme, roughly chopped

Generous pinch of cayenne pepper (more if desired)

3 medium-size baking potatoes, peeled and very thinly sliced, using a mandoline or sharp knife

Finely chopped fresh chives or parsley sprigs for garnish (optional)

This is one of our favorite dishes that our dad makes quite regularly over the winter months, though he makes it with real wheat-flour pie crusts. We shed quite a few tears when we realized we couldn't partake of his pot pie deliciousness any longer. So we embarked on a mission to create a gluten-free version, and the result is as comforting as slipping on a big old sweater on a cold night. The other result to all our taste testing and mastering of this deliciousness was our jeans' not fitting so well! This is a surprisingly easy dish to put together and will impress even the pickiest of eaters. We've used Lyonnaise, or very thinly sliced, potatoes as our topping instead of the more traditional pie crust. What can we say—we like shaking things up and going against the conventional grain! You're left with a scrumptious dish that's layered with many different textures and aromatic flavors. Feel free to gather round the fireplace and get cozy with this one.

SERVES 6 TO 8

STEPS

❶ Place the diced chicken in a small bowl and toss with the seasoning to coat thoroughly.

❷ In a medium-size skillet or sauté pan, heat the olive oil over medium heat. Add the chicken and sauté, turning the pieces occasionally, until cooked through, about 8 minutes. Set aside.

❸ In a medium-size (6-quart) stockpot or Dutch oven, melt the butter over medium heat. Add the onions, celery, garlic, salt, and black pepper and cook until the vegetables begin to soften, about 3 to 4 minutes.

❹ Stir in the flour blend to make a blond roux and cook an additional 4 minutes, stirring constantly.

❺ Add the chicken stock and wine, if using, and bring to a gentle boil over high heat. Make sure the flour from the roux and the liquids are well incorporated. Once the sauce is boiling and bubbling, reduce the heat to medium low and simmer until the sauce thickens, about 5 minutes.

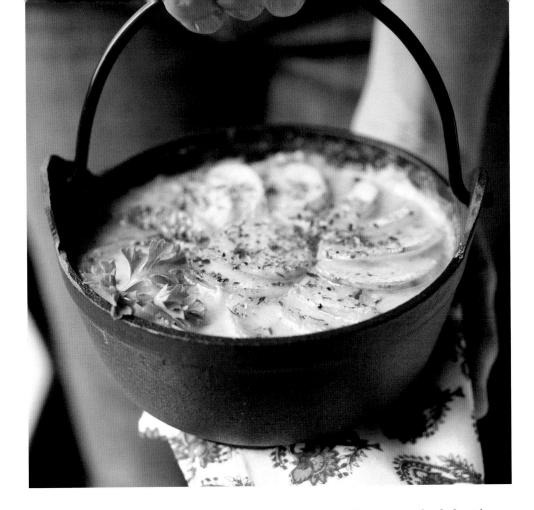

6 Add the half-and-half, stir well, and cook another 4 minutes.

7 Add the carrots, peas, cooked chicken, thyme, cayenne pepper, and a bit more salt and black pepper to taste. Stir the mixture very well. Remove from the heat to cool slightly.

8 Preheat the oven to 375°F.

9 Spread the filling mixture out evenly in an ovenproof casserole dish or simply pour the filling into a Dutch oven.

10 Layer the sliced potatoes over the top of the mixture to create a crust, starting at the center and working your way outward until all the potato slices have been used. (Some of the potatoes may sink into the filling mixture; this is fine. Just keep layering.)

11 Season the potatoes well with salt and black pepper and bake for 40 to 45 minutes, or until the potatoes are cooked through. Once the potatoes are golden brown, about halfway through cooking, cover the dish with aluminum foil to prevent the potatoes from burning. Please note that, depending on the thickness of the sliced potatoes, you may need to adjust your cooking time up to 1 hour.

12 If desired, garnish the top of the pie with a sprinkling of chopped chives or a parsley sprig. Serve while hot.

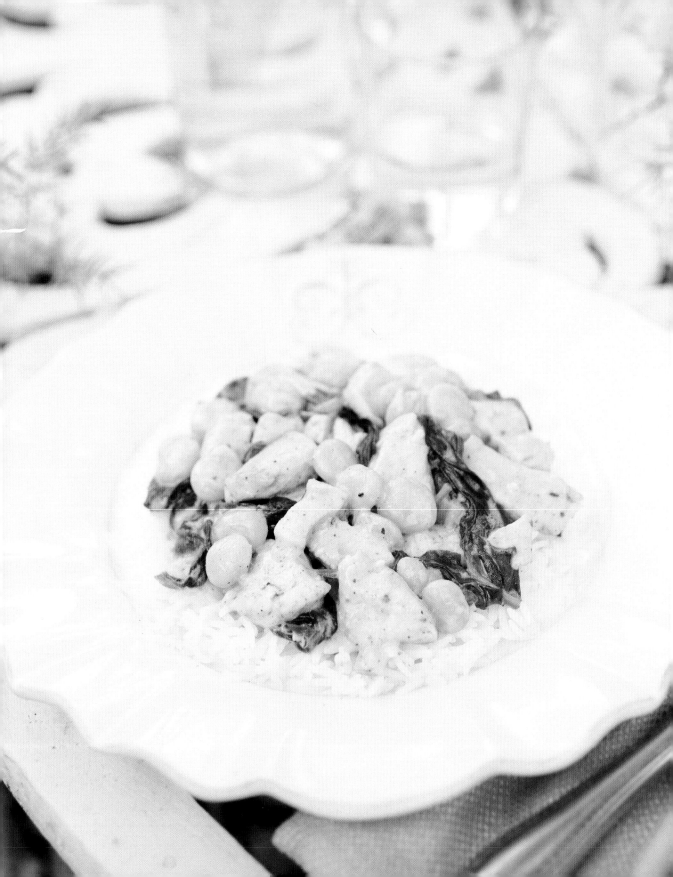

dijon chicken
with spinach *and* lima beans

INGREDIENTS

¾ pound boneless, skinless chicken breasts, diced into bite-size chunks

1½ teaspoons Emeril's Original Essence Seasoning or Cajun seasoning of your choice

2 tablespoons olive oil

2 cloves garlic, minced

½ cup lima beans, canned or frozen, drained if canned

4 green onions, thinly sliced diagonally, white and green parts kept separate

Salt and black pepper to taste

1 cup (8 ounces) crème fraîche

2 tablespoons Dijon mustard

4 cups spinach leaves, washed and patted dry

Large pinch of ground or freshly grated nutmeg

Cooked gluten-free pasta or rice, for serving

Freshly grated Parmesan cheese, for serving (optional)

Try shaking up your chicken routine with this zingy one-pot meal. This succulent chicken dish is full of tangy creaminess from the Dijon mustard and crème fraîche, fortified with a healthy helping of spinach and then accented with the flavor of the lima beans. In our opinion, lima beans are highly underrated! It's a shame limas have such a bad rep, because they are packed full of heart-healthy fiber and protein. This dish will show you how delicious they can be. Even your kids will want seconds. You should be able to find canned or frozen lima beans at your local grocery store, but you really need the crème fraîche for the dish and its sauce to work (see the Beef Stroganoff with Rice Noodles recipe on page 164 for more information about crème fraîche). Serve this versatile midweek dish over anything you like—steamed rice, your favorite gluten-free pasta, or even our Sour Cream and Chive Mash (page 114). Go, Mr. Lima Bean, go!

SERVES 2 TO 4

STEPS

❶ Place the chicken in a medium-size bowl and toss with the Essence Seasoning to coat thoroughly.

❷ In a large, deep-sided sauté pan over medium-high heat, heat the oil.

❸ Add the seasoned chicken pieces and garlic and sauté, stirring frequently, until the chicken is fully cooked through and a nice golden color, about 6 minutes, depending on the size of the pieces.

❹ Turn the heat down to medium and add the lima beans, white part of the green onions, and salt and pepper to taste. Stir well and sauté gently for 5 minutes.

❺ Turn the heat down to low and stir in the crème fraîche and Dijon mustard. Add the remaining green onion, the spinach, nutmeg, and more salt and pepper to taste. Stir well and simmer for 2 to 3 minutes to allow the spinach to wilt.

❻ Turn off the heat and serve immediately over cooked pasta or rice, topped, if desired, with a generous sprinkling of grated Parmesan cheese.

slow-cooked rosemary chicken
with apples *and* fennel

INGREDIENTS

1 tablespoon unsalted butter

2 medium-size or 3 small apples of your choice, peeled, cored, and sliced (enough to make 3 cups)

1 large bulb fennel, trimmed of tough outer layer and sliced lengthwise (about 2 cups)

1 large yellow onion, sliced

2 pounds chicken, skinless or skin on, pieces or boneless breasts

2½ tablespoons chopped fresh rosemary leaves

1 teaspoon celery salt

½ teaspoon salt

Black pepper to taste

1 cup chicken or vegetable stock

2 cups cooked wild rice, for serving

Get out your slow cooker and dust it off, people, because this is a fantastic one-pot meal everyone will adore. This warm and comforting dish is a perfect autumn meal, when apples and fennel are both in season and readily available. Some people can be a bit intimidated when it comes to working with fennel, but the aniseed, licorice-like flavor adds a wonderful depth to this dish. Just peel the outer layer and chop off the stalk and sprout bits, and the rest is usable and scrumptious. The chicken will be so tender, don't be surprised if you can eat this dish with just a spoon. To complete the recipe, we've recommended serving the chicken on top of cooked wild rice, which adds an earthy nuttiness. But feel free to serve this with any rice you prefer. Pears work well in place of the apples, too, for a slight variation. Jilly prefers this recipe using bone-in chicken pieces, whereas Jessie likes to use boneless chicken breasts. It's entirely up to you, though if using bone-in cuts, be mindful of bones when eating, especially if you're feeding little ones!

SERVES 4

STEPS

1 Put the butter in the bottom of either a Crock-Pot/slow cooker or a Dutch oven. If using a Dutch oven, preheat the oven to 350°F.

2 Arrange the apples, fennel, and onion slices over the bottom of the pan.

3 Lay the chicken pieces on top. Sprinkle on the rosemary, celery salt, and a generous bit of salt and pepper.

4 Pour the stock over the chicken, cover with a lid, and cook as follows. If using a Crock-Pot/slow cooker, cook on low for 6 to 8 hours or high for 3 to 4 hours. If using a Dutch oven, cook in the 350°F oven for 3 to 4 hours, or until the chicken is falling apart.

5 Serve over cooked wild rice.

roasted rosemary chicken
with veggies

INGREDIENTS

2 medium-size red potatoes, cut into bite-size pieces (about 3 cups)

1 medium-size yellow onion, sliced (about 1½ cups)

2 medium-size carrots, peeled and sliced (about 1 cup)

¼ cup olive oil, plus additional for coating the chicken

4 teaspoons very finely chopped fresh rosemary leaves

½ teaspoon salt, plus more to taste

Black pepper to taste

½ cup chicken stock

1 lemon

4 boneless, skinless chicken breasts, trimmed of fat

Rosemary is something you can always find growing to excess in Jessie's garden. Her oldest son, Jude, helps her cut the pieces off the plant so she can use them for dinner, especially in this tasty chicken dish. Though this is a straightforward recipe, it is very delicious and certainly very good for you. Be sure to roast the veggies alone first so they have time to become tender without drying the chicken out.

SERVES 4

STEPS

1 Preheat the oven to 400°F.

2 In a medium-size bowl, toss the potatoes, onion, and carrots with the ¼ cup olive oil, 2 teaspoons of the rosemary, ½ teaspoon salt, and black pepper to taste until the vegetables are thoroughly coated and the ingredients are evenly distributed.

3 Make a layer of the vegetables in a 13 × 9–inch baking dish. Pour in the chicken stock. Slice the lemon in half and squeeze the juice over the whole pan. Bake for 20 minutes.

4 While the vegetables are baking, brush the chicken breasts with olive oil just to coat. Season with additional salt and pepper as desired and sprinkle with the remaining 2 teaspoons rosemary.

5 Carefully remove the baking dish from the oven. Place the seasoned chicken breasts on top of the bed of vegetables. Cover the entire dish with foil. Return the dish to the oven for another 20 to 30 minutes, or until the chicken breasts are cooked through (internal temperature of 165°F).

6 Remove from the oven and serve immediately.

beef *and* red wine casserole

½ cup gluten-free all-purpose flour blend (we've used Arrowhead Mills Gluten Free All Purpose Baking Mix)

1 tablespoon Emeril's Original Essence Seasoning or Steak Rub Seasoning, or Cajun or steak rub seasoning of your choice

3 sprigs fresh rosemary, leaves only, finely chopped

2 pounds beef chuck or stewing steak, trimmed and cubed

¼ cup olive oil

1½ cups peeled, quartered shallots

2 small cloves garlic, minced

1 cup red wine (we've used Shiraz)

2 cups plus 1 tablespoon beef stock

1 tablespoon cornstarch

2 tablespoons plus 1½ teaspoons tomato paste

6 sprigs fresh thyme, leaves only, chopped

1 teaspoon celery salt

Salt and black pepper to taste

2 medium baking potatoes, such as Idaho variety, cut into bite-size chunks (about 2 cups)

4 medium-size carrots, peeled and chopped (about 2 cups)

3 large stalks celery, trimmed and cut into chunks (about 1½ cups)

1 bay leaf

This is the gluten-free take on one of our mother's specialties, a fantastic one-pot meal perfect for warming you up on those cold winter nights. Even better, as with most one-pot meals, it requires minimal cleanup. If you want to, you can use a Crock-Pot, which happens to be one of Jessie's favorite kitchen tools, instead. Simply follow the instructions to step 9; then place all contents into the Crock-Pot, and cook it slow and low, baby, for 6 to 8 hours. We've used Shiraz wine for this recipe, but feel free to use anything you would enjoy drinking. That's Jilly's motto: a lil' splash for the casserole, a lil' splash in a wine glass—it's a win-win situation. Our Zucchini and Polenta Fritters on page 30 make an excellent accompaniment to this hearty casserole, or serve with your favorite brand of gluten-free bread or rolls. We really love Against The Grain Gourmet's baguettes.

SERVES 4 TO 6

STEPS

❶ In a medium-size bowl, combine the flour blend, Essence Seasoning, and rosemary and stir with a fork to mix together.

❷ Place the steak chunks in the bowl and dredge the meat until all sides are well covered. Put aside.

❸ Preheat the oven to 300°F.

❹ In a medium-size (6-quart) Dutch oven over medium heat, heat 2 tablespoons of the olive oil. If you are using a Crock-Pot, perform steps 4 to 9 in a pan on the stovetop, and then transfer the contents to the Crock-Pot.

❺ Add the shallots and garlic and sauté until slightly softened, about 4 minutes.

❻ Using a slotted spoon, remove the shallots and garlic to a large bowl. Set aside.

❼ Add the remaining 2 tablespoons oil to the Dutch oven and heat over medium-high heat. Add the meat, in batches, and sauté until just browned on all sides.

❽ Remove each batch of meat and place it in the bowl with the shallots and set aside.

9 Turn the heat under the Dutch oven down to low and add the red wine and 2 cups of the beef stock. Stir well, making sure to loosen any browned bits on the bottom of the pan.

10 In a small bowl or measuring cup, mix the remaining stock and the cornstarch until the cornstarch is fully dissolved.

11 Add this cornstarch mixture, the tomato paste, thyme, celery salt, and salt and pepper to the Dutch oven. Stir well.

12 Return the meat and shallots to the Dutch oven, stir well, and turn off the heat.

13 Add the potatoes, carrots, celery, and bay leaf. Stir together and season with more pepper.

14 Cover with a lid and cook for 2 to 2½ hours in the oven, or until the meat is very tender. If using a Crock-Pot, set pot to the 6- or 8-hour setting and cook.

15 Remove the bay leaf before serving.

beef stroganoff *with* rice noodles

INGREDIENTS

1 pound sirloin steak, trimmed of fat and cut into long, thin slices

1 teaspoon Emeril's Original Essence Seasoning or Cajun seasoning of your choice

Pepper, preferably freshly cracked black pepper, to taste

2 tablespoons unsalted butter

1 small yellow onion, halved and thinly sliced

1 small red onion, halved and thinly sliced

2 cloves garlic, minced

1 cup sliced cremini, or baby bella, mushrooms (about 2 ounces, brushed clean)

⅓ cup dry white wine

1 cup frozen peas

⅔ cup crème fraîche

1 tablespoon Dijon mustard

Salt to taste

1 tablespoon chopped fresh parsley

1 tablespoon chopped fresh thyme leaves

1 package (8 ounces) rice noodles, cooked as directed

This dish was created as an ode to our amazing and wonderful grandpa Kief. He can't get enough of a good beef stroganoff. For him to give us his seal of approval—which was a very energetic "Mmmmm"—we must be doing something right. You can substitute cooking sherry for the dry white wine; just remember to *always* cook with wine you wouldn't actually mind drinking yourself. Very important! This dish contains a key ingredient, crème fraîche, which is a French cultured cream, similar to sour cream in taste but with a higher percentage of butterfat content. The butterfat makes it perfect for cooked sauces because it won't curdle or break. If you can't find crème fraîche in your local grocery store, try your specialty food or cheese store. It's a wonderful and naturally gluten-free thickener for sauces. We suggest serving this over thick pad thai–cut rice noodles to soak up all the delicious juices. Slice the beef to your preferred thickness and feel free to use any cut of steak you like.

SERVES 4

STEPS

❶ Toss the sliced steak with the Essence Seasoning and a generous amount of black pepper in a medium-size bowl and set aside.

❷ In a large (3-quart) skillet with deep sides, melt the butter over medium heat.

❸ Add the onions and garlic and sauté until the onions are slightly browned and softened, about 5 minutes.

❹ Add the steak pieces and brown on all sides until cooked through.

❺ Add the mushrooms to the skillet and cook for 4 minutes.

❻ Add the wine. Increase the heat to medium high and bring the mixture to a gentle boil. Cook until the liquid has reduced, about 4 to 5 minutes.

❼ Add the frozen peas, crème fraîche, mustard, and salt and pepper to taste and stir well.

❽ Turn the heat down to low and let simmer for 5 minutes.

❾ Stir in the parsley and thyme and cook another 4 to 5 minutes. The peas should be warmed through.

❿ Serve immediately over the prepared rice noodles.

chicken fried rice

INGREDIENTS

1 cup rice

2 cups chicken stock

1 cup thinly sliced carrot

2 large eggs, beaten

2 tablespoons olive oil

1 cup diced yellow onion

2 teaspoons minced garlic

¼ cup diced celery

2 boneless, skinless chicken breasts, trimmed of fat and diced

Salt to taste

¼ teaspoon black pepper

1 cup trimmed and diced snow peas (about 4 ounces)

2 to 3 tablespoons gluten-free soy sauce

1 teaspoon toasted sesame oil

Even before Jessie was diagnosed with gluten intolerance, she made this meal weekly. It is full of healthy veggies, protein, and heart-friendly oils. Feel free to adjust the soy sauce and sesame oil to suit your preference. A brief word of warning: be sure that you are using gluten-free soy sauce since many popular brands do contain gluten!

SERVES 4

STEPS

1 Following directions on the box or bag, prepare 4 servings of rice in a small saucepan. However, cook the rice in the chicken stock instead of water. Set aside once cooked.

2 Bring a small saucepan of water to a boil. Blanch the carrots in the boiling water, draining them after about 1 minute. Run them under cold water for about 1 minute to stop the cooking process. Set aside.

3 In a small nonstick skillet over medium heat, scramble the eggs and set aside.

4 In a large nonstick skillet over medium heat, heat the olive oil. Add the onion and sauté until it just begins to soften, about 3 minutes.

5 Add the garlic, celery, chicken, salt to taste, and pepper. Continue cooking, stirring frequently, for another 5 minutes.

6 Add the carrots and snow peas and continue cooking another 5 to 7 minutes, or until the chicken pieces are cooked through.

7 Once the chicken pieces are cooked, fold in the eggs. Add the cooked rice, soy sauce, and sesame oil. Stir until all the ingredients are evenly distributed. Cook for another 2 to 3 minutes, stirring frequently.

8 Take off the heat and serve immediately.

spinach *and* ricotta lasagna

INGREDIENTS

3 tablespoons olive oil

1 medium-size yellow onion, chopped

2 cloves garlic, minced

7 cups fresh spinach leaves, washed and patted dry (about 10 to 12 ounces)

1 container (15 ounces) ricotta cheese

1 teaspoon Emeril's Italian Seasoning or Italian seasoning of your choice

½ teaspoon celery salt

Salt and black pepper to taste

3 cups tomato-based pasta sauce of choice

1 box (16 sheets total) no-boil gluten-free/wheat-free lasagna sheets

¼ cup freshly grated Parmesan cheese

Talk about a seriously delicious and gorgeous vegetarian dish, satisfying enough for even the hungriest of giants! Earthy spinach and creamy ricotta make this a culinary marriage made in Heaven. Plus, who ever knew that eating a big ol' plate of lasagna could be so good for you? With the vitamin C–packed spinach and the calcium-packed ricotta, this dish packs a one-two punch. You should be able to find gluten-free lasagna sheets at most of your local grocery or health food shops. Promise us you'll give this recipe a try for your next Sunday family dinner and we'll promise *you* that everyone is going to love it! Don't forget—you can use the homemade sauce from our Spaghetti with Meatballs recipe (page 149) for this, or any store-bought variety you like. Eat up, everyone!

SERVES 8 TO 10

STEPS

❶ Preheat the oven to 400°F.

❷ In a large (3-quart) sauté pan heat the olive oil over medium heat. Add the onion and garlic and sauté for 4 minutes.

❸ Add the spinach, in batches, to the pan until it has all been included and is wilted, about 3 minutes.

❹ Add the ricotta, Italian seasoning, celery salt, and salt and pepper, stirring well to incorporate all the spinach with the ricotta and seasonings. Turn off the heat.

❺ In a 13 × 9–inch lasagna pan or baking dish, start to assemble the lasagna: ladle 2 spoonfuls of pasta sauce into the dish and spread evenly to cover the bottom. Continue assembling the lasagna in steps 6 through 9.

❻ Make a single layer of 4 uncooked lasagna sheets on top of the sauce on the bottom of the pan.

❼ Layer 4 generous spoonfuls of the spinach-ricotta mixture over the sheets, spreading the mixture out as best as possible to cover the sheets.

❽ Top with one-third of the remaining sauce, one-quarter of the Parmesan cheese, and another layer of lasagna sheets.

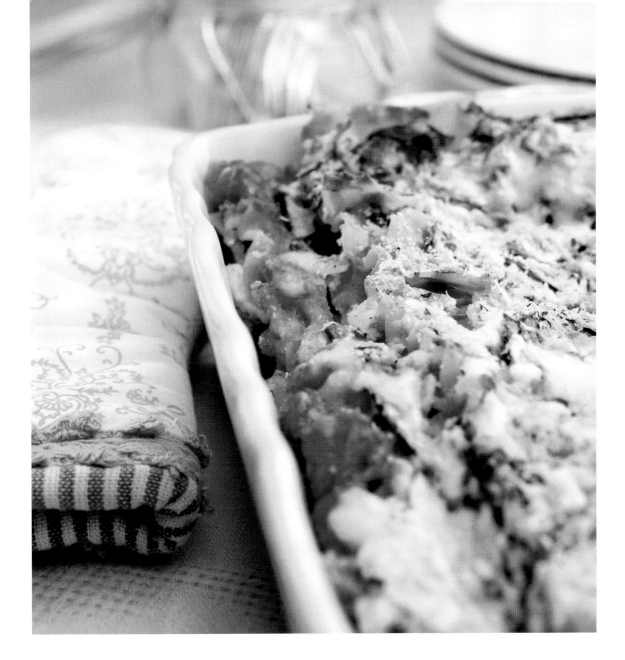

9 Repeat steps 7 and 8 twice to make two more layers with all of the ingredients. Then make your final layer, which consists of lasagna sheets, the remaining spinach-ricotta mixture, and the remaining Parmesan cheese.

10 Bake uncovered for an initial 30 minutes before covering with foil and baking another 15 to 20 minutes, or until the lasagna sheets are cooked through.

11 Let stand 4 to 5 minutes before serving.

italian sausage, basil, *and* mushroom lasagna

INGREDIENTS

3 tablespoons olive oil

2 cloves garlic, minced

4 gluten-free spicy Italian sausages, pork or turkey (about 1 pound)

2 cups roughly chopped cremini, or baby bella, mushrooms (about 4 ounces), brushed clean

1 medium-size yellow onion, chopped

1 tablespoon Emeril's Italian Seasoning or Italian seasoning of your choice

1 tablespoon celery salt

Pinch of crushed red pepper flakes (optional)

Salt and black pepper to taste

3 cups tomato-based pasta sauce of choice

1 box (16 sheets total) no-boil gluten-free/wheat-free lasagna sheets

⅓ cup freshly grated Parmesan cheese

2 large handfuls fresh basil leaves, washed and patted dry

This is a delicious dish the whole family will enjoy, celiac disease or not! Italian food is one of our absolute favorites, but when we were first diagnosed, it was devastating to think of never again being able to enjoy a homemade lasagna, ravioli, or even hot brick-oven pizza. However, gluten-free pastas and pizza bases are tastier than ever before and are now more readily available. This is a fabulous dish to take to a new mother, a neighbor, or even your friend's next dinner party. You can bake it in a regular lasagna pan, though we prefer to use a large clear Pyrex dish so you can see all the beautiful layers of basil. Use any store-bought gluten-free lasagna sheets you like; we've used a corn-based brand.

Feel free to also use any type of sausage you prefer: pork, turkey or none at all for a delectable vegetarian meal. Just be sure to always check your labels. Wheat flour is often used to bulk up store-bought sausages. You can use the homemade red sauce from our Spaghetti with Meatballs recipe on page 149 or any store-bought brand you like. This lasagna makes a gorgeous dish not only for the eyes, but also for the tummy. We know you're going to love this!

SERVES 8

STEPS

❶ Preheat the oven to 400°F.

❷ In a large sauté pan over medium heat, heat the oil. Add the garlic and sauté for 3 minutes, stirring occasionally so the garlic doesn't burn.

❸ On a cutting board or clean work surface, cut the sausages open lengthwise with a knife. Free the meat from the casings and crumble the meat into the pan. Dispose of the casings.

❹ Cook the meat until fully cooked and browned, about 8 to 10 minutes, making sure to crumble with a wooden spoon while cooking.

❺ Drain any excess fat from the pan, though if using lean meat, there shouldn't be much.

❻ Add the mushrooms, onion, Italian seasoning, celery salt, crushed red pepper flakes if using, and salt and black pepper to taste. Stir well.

7 Turn the heat down to medium low. Add the pasta sauce and simmer for 5 minutes, stirring frequently.

8 Turn off the heat and set aside.

9 Now assemble the lasagna, using the same alternating steps you would in making any lasagna. Start by ladling 2 heaping spoonfuls of the sauce and meat mixture into your pan, spreading it evenly to cover the bottom.

10 Make a single layer of 4 uncooked lasagna sheets on top of the sauce. Ladle 2 more heaping spoonfuls of sauce on top of the sheets, spreading evenly. Sprinkle a heaping tablespoonful of grated Parmesan cheese over the sauce.

11 Add a layer of fresh basil leaves, figuring roughly 4 leaves per lasagna sheet.

12 Repeat this layering process three times: sheets (4 per layer), sauce, cheese, and then basil. Sprinkle with top layer of basil and the remaining cheese.

13 Cover the pan loosely with aluminum foil to prevent the basil from burning or drying out.

14 Bake for 35 to 45 minutes, or until the lasagna sheets are cooked through and soft.

15 Let stand for 4 to 5 minutes before serving.

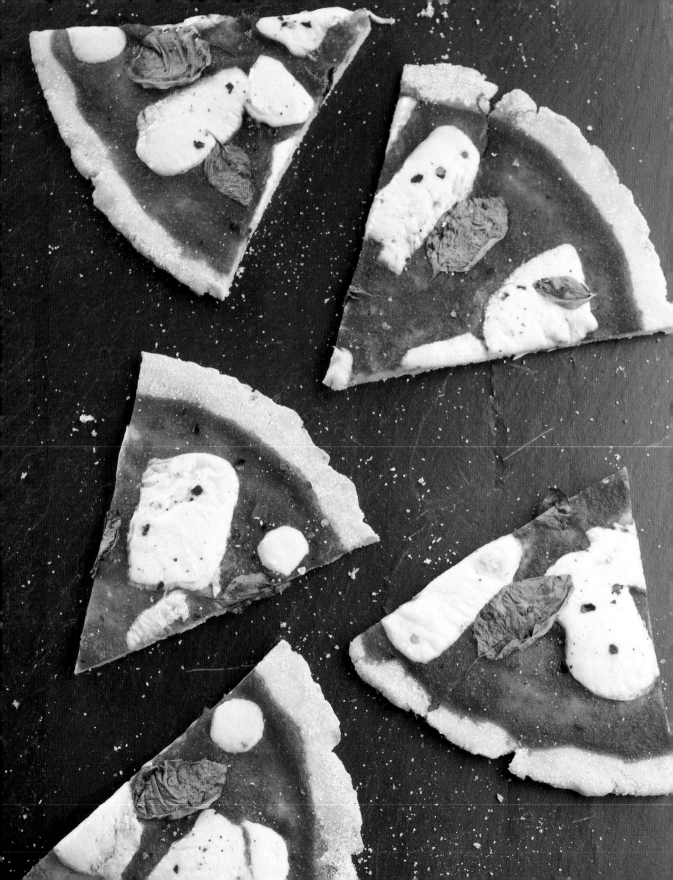

emeril's gluten-free pizza

INGREDIENTS

1 cup warm water (no hotter than 110°F)

2 tablespoons active dry yeast

1 tablespoon sugar

Vegetable oil spray

2 cups white rice flour

½ cup soy flour

⅔ cup instant nonfat dry milk powder

2 cups tapioca flour

3 teaspoons xanthan gum

1 teaspoon salt

3 tablespoons olive oil

½ cup hot water

4 large eggs, whites only, at room temperature

Favorite sauce and topping ingredients

For us, pizza is just one of those comfort foods that we must eat on a regular basis. A nice spicy sauce, fresh toppings, and, of course, a delicious crust make pizza a craving-quenching treat we love. This recipe from our dad produces a terrific gluten-free crust from scratch—no premixed flour blends here! You can top this pizza crust with any and all of your favorite toppings. White sauce or red, sausage or shrimp, this crust will complement them all!

YIELDS ENOUGH DOUGH FOR TWO 14- TO 16-INCH PIZZAS

STEPS

❶ Preheat the oven to 400°F.

❷ Combine the 1 cup warm water, 2 tablespoons active dry yeast, and sugar. Set aside until the yeast is foamy, about 5 minutes.

❸ Liberally spray two large baking pans with nonstick cooking spray and set aside.

❹ Combine the white rice flour, soy flour, milk powder, tapioca flour, xanthan gum, and salt in the bowl of a standing mixer with a paddle attached. Mix on low until the flour is well incorporated. Little by little add the olive oil and the ½ cup of hot water.

❺ Slowly drizzle in the egg whites until the mixture is fully incorporated. Add the yeast mixture and combine. Increase the speed to high and mix for 4 minutes.

❻ Remove the dough from the mixing bowl and evenly divide into two balls. Place one of the dough balls onto each pan. Using lightly greased hands, gently press each portion of dough into a 14- to 16-inch circle about ¼ inch thick, leaving the dough around the edges a bit thicker. Set aside for 10 minutes to rise.

❼ Place the dough into the oven and let cook for 5 minutes.

❽ Remove from the oven and top with your favorite sauce and ingredients.

❾ Place back into the oven and continue to cook until the crust is golden brown and crispy, 10 to 12 minutes longer. (Note: it is important that the baking pan is liberally greased; otherwise the dough will stick. If this happens, use a flat metal spatula to separate the dough from the baking pan.)

chickpea *and* ginger curry

INGREDIENTS

¼ cup vegetable oil

1 large yellow onion, chopped

1½ teaspoons grated fresh ginger

2 cloves garlic, minced

Pinch of crushed red pepper flakes, or to taste

1½ cups sliced cremini, or baby bella, mushrooms (about 3 ounces), brushed clean

1½ cups frozen green peas

Pinch of salt, or to taste

2 tablespoons Indian curry paste, mild or Madras (we've used Patak's brand)

2 teaspoons garam masala

¾ teaspoon ground turmeric

2 teaspoons granulated sugar, or to taste

1 medium-size tomato, cut into wedges

1 cup tomato sauce

1 cup (8 ounces) crème fraîche

1 can (7 ounces) chickpeas or chana, drained well

⅓ cup roughly chopped fresh cilantro leaves

Cooked basmati rice, for serving (optional)

Jilly wasn't introduced to Indian cuisine until she moved to London. Now it has become one of her most favorite styles of food, and she can't seem to make it through a whole week without giving in to her hankering for "a good cuzza." She loves curries for their sheer versatility and the amazing layers of flavors and spices. One bite and your whole palate is dancing with sweet, spice, tang…ahhh. You can use any vegetables or proteins you like. Or keep it completely vegetarian with paneer or chickpeas, also known as *chana*. The possibilities are endless, and so is the flavor. Indians say you eat with your eyes, not your stomach. Needless to say, their food reflects that belief by being vibrant and rich in colors, spices, and smells. It's a delight for all of your senses. Our hope is that this humble curry may even lead some of our readers into the love and appreciation of Indian food and flavors.

Please note: you should be able to find Indian curry paste in the ethnic aisle of your local grocery store. Use a mild paste if you're not used to heat or Madras paste if you can handle heat. Avoid vindaloo curry paste, as it will be too hot for this dish. If you find the curry too spicy for your liking after cooking, add more sugar.

SERVES 4

STEPS

❶ In a large (3-quart) saucepan over medium heat, heat the oil. Add the onion, ginger, garlic, and crushed red pepper flakes and sauté until the onion is slightly softened, about 4 minutes.

❷ Add the mushrooms, peas, and a pinch of salt, stir well, and cook another 4 minutes.

❸ Add the curry paste, garam masala, turmeric, sugar, and tomato wedges. Stir to coat the vegetables with the seasonings.

❹ Turn the heat down to low and simmer for 5 minutes.

❺ Add the tomato sauce, crème fraîche, chickpeas, and cilantro. Stir well.

❻ Allow to simmer, uncovered, for 30 minutes longer.

❼ Re-season with more salt, sugar, or crushed red pepper flakes, if desired. Turn off the heat and serve, if desired, over boiled or steamed basmati rice.

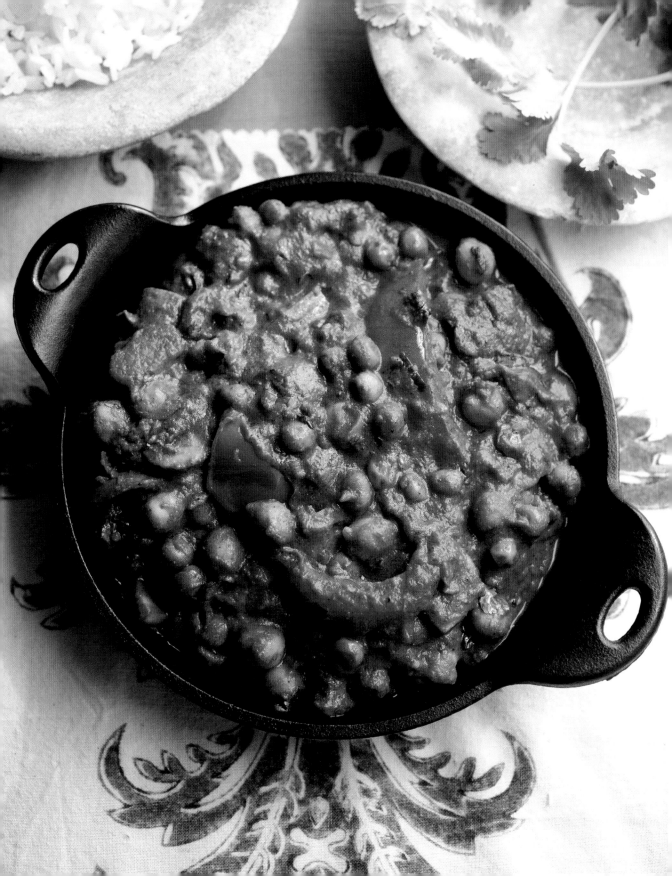

spicy szechuan chicken *with* cashews, broccoli, *and* green onions

INGREDIENTS

3 boneless, skinless chicken breasts, cut into bite-size pieces (about 1 inch each)

1 large egg white

6 teaspoons cornstarch

2½ cups broccoli florets

⅔ cup water

2 tablespoons gluten-free soy sauce or tamari

2 tablespoons vegetable or sunflower oil

½ cup cashews or peanuts, roughly chopped

1 teaspoon crushed red pepper flakes

Pinch of salt

2 tablespoons toasted sesame oil

2 teaspoons granulated sugar

2 teaspoons white wine or rice vinegar

4 green onions, thinly sliced

This is a delicious gluten-free take on one of our favorite dishes, kung pao chicken. Unfortunately for celiacs, Chinese restaurants in the US tend to bread and deep-fry their chicken for this dish. The devilish wheat flour is also frequently used to thicken up all those tasty sauces, which usually contain traditional soy sauce—another big no-no. But have no fear, for you can make even tastier, and healthier, Chinese food at home! We know you will love this fresh and vibrant dish full of the spicy tang and crunch kung pao is known for. We recommend serving it alongside a hot steamy bowl of our Sesame Stir-Fried Rice (recipe on page 121). Or try serving with simple boiled rice to really let the dish be the star. Please note that the chicken will need to marinate for 1 to 3 hours, so you'll have to plan ahead of time.

SERVES 4

STEPS

1 In a medium-size bowl, combine the chicken pieces, egg white, and 4 teaspoons of the cornstarch. Stir well to thoroughly coat the chicken.

2 Cover with cling film and chill in the refrigerator for at least 1 hour, but not exceeding 3.

3 In a medium-size saucepan of boiling salted water, blanch the broccoli florets for 2 to 3 minutes.

4 While the broccoli is cooking, fill a medium-size bowl with water and ice cubes. Drain the broccoli and shock in the ice-water bath for 1 minute to stop it from cooking further. (You want the florets to maintain their bite.) Drain again and set aside.

5 When the chicken has marinated sufficiently, take it out of the refrigerator.

6 In a small bowl, stir the remaining 2 teaspoons cornstarch, the water, and the soy sauce to mix well. Set aside.

7 In a medium-size sauté pan or wok over medium heat, heat the vegetable oil. Add the chopped nuts, the red pepper flakes, and a pinch of salt and sauté until the nuts are lightly browned and toasted, about 1 to 2 minutes.

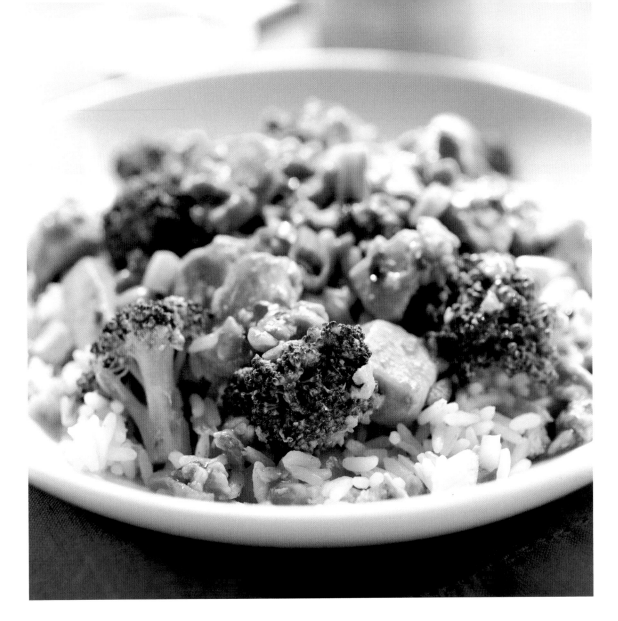

8 Remove the nuts to a bowl and set aside.

9 Add the marinated chicken, sesame oil, and sugar to the pan, and stir-fry until the chicken is cooked through and golden brown, about 8 to 9 minutes, depending on the size of the pieces.

10 Add the vinegar, stir, and allow to evaporate, about 1 minute, before stirring in the reserved nuts, the broccoli, the soy sauce mixture, and the green onions (reserving a few slices for garnish, if desired). Season with a bit more salt and stir well.

11 As soon as the sauce has thickened, about 3 minutes, remove from the heat and serve immediately, garnished with a sprinkling of sliced green onion, if desired.

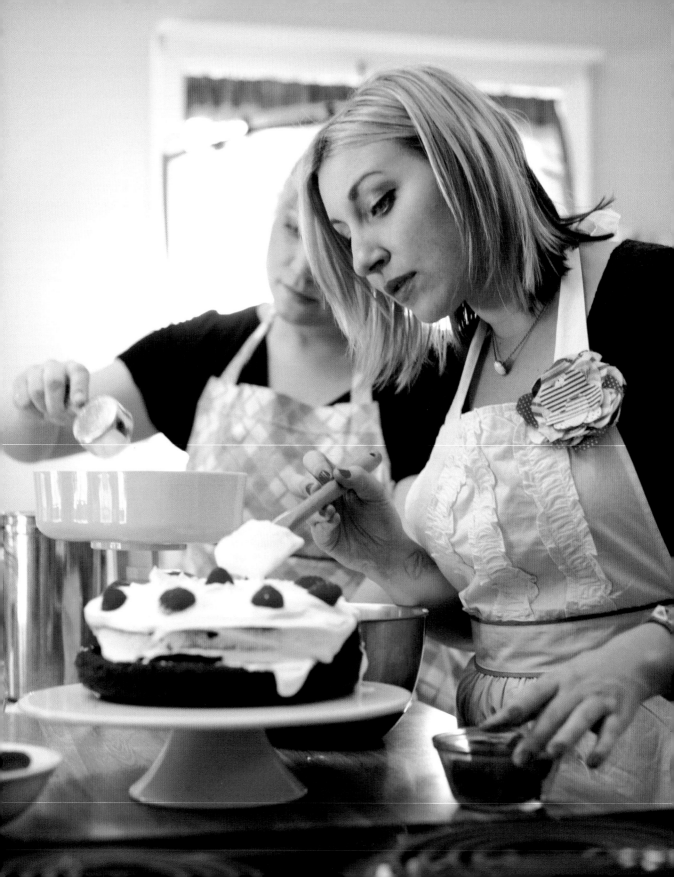

desserts

There's not much more we need to say about desserts other than…
yum! Both of us are dessert-aholics, to say the least. Our preferences
run the gamut from decadent chocolate indulgences to home-style
fruit deliciousness. Warm or cold, cake or muffin, fruit or nuts,
there are recipes here to hit everyone's sweet spot. Many of these
are gluten-free versions of our personal favorites, inspired by
family, mentors, and friends. They are regular features on our home
tables for holidays, birthdays (Jessie's husband *loves* the Classic
Key Lime Pie for his birthday), or any day. We sincerely hope you
can incorporate many of these tasty desserts in your own family
traditions just as we have. Enjoy!

classic key lime pie

INGREDIENTS

crust

2½ cups gluten-free cookies, ginger or graham cracker, if possible

4 tablespoons (½ stick) unsalted butter, melted

filling

2 cans (14 ounces each) light condensed milk

2 large eggs

1 cup fresh lime juice, key lime if available

1 cup sour cream

2 tablespoons confectioner's sugar (powdered sugar)

1 tablespoon freshly grated lime zest

Thin lime slices, for garnish (optional)

Jilly learned to make this recipe while working at her dad's first restaurant, Emeril's. She used to work there over summer breaks for experience and, of course, extra pocket money. One summer, she was lucky enough to work with Mr. Lou, one of the most amazing pastry chefs and people she has ever had the pleasure of knowing. Although he rarely let anyone write down his recipes, this gluten-free version of key lime pie is as close to his original as Jilly could get. This one is for you, Mr. Lou!

SERVES 8

STEPS

crust

1 Roughly break up the cookies and place them in the bowl of a food processor along with the melted butter. Pulse until the mixture forms crumbs.

2 Using your fingertips, press the crumb mixture firmly over the bottom of a 9-inch deep-dish pie plate or cake pan. Spread out and pat evenly until a bottom crust is achieved.

3 Place the crust in the refrigerator to set for 30 minutes.

filling

1 Preheat the oven to 325°F.

2 In a large bowl, combine the condensed milk, eggs, and lime juice and whisk until well blended.

3 Remove the pie crust from the refrigerator and pour in the filling mixture. Place in the oven and bake for 20 minutes, or until the center of the pie is not jiggly.

4 Remove the pie from the oven and allow it to cool until it reaches room temperature. Then place the pie in the refrigerator for 2 hours to allow it to set.

(recipe continues)

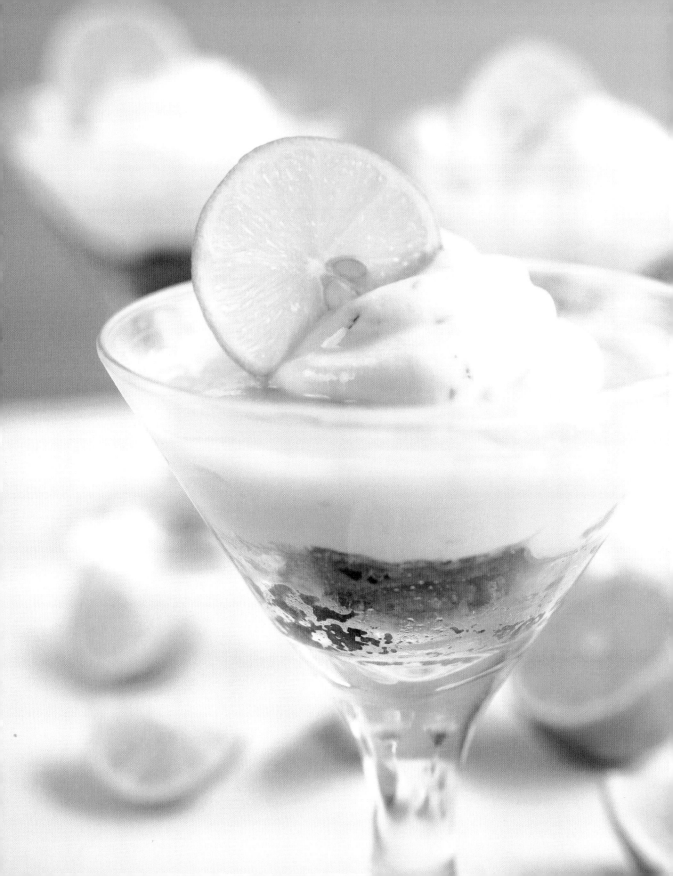

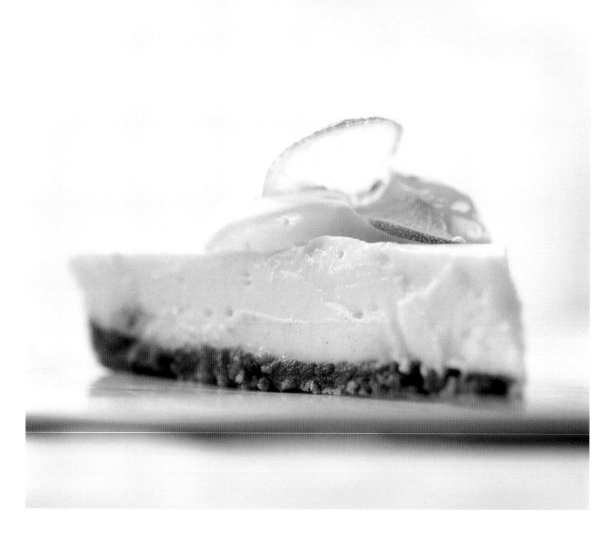

STEPS (CONT.)

5 Once the pie is chilled, combine the sour cream, confectioner's sugar, and half the lime zest in a medium-size bowl and mix well.

6 Spread this mixture evenly over the top of the pie. Sprinkle the remaining lime zest on top. If desired, garnish the pie with thin lime slices as well.

7 Store the pie in the refrigerator until ready to serve.

note: After the pie has been baked and chilled, you can change up the presentation, if you want. Carefully scoop out individual portions of the crust and filling and transfer them to whatever individual serving vessels you prefer. Then, once you make the topping in Step 5, spread it on each portion and serve.

chocolate raspberry bars

INGREDIENTS

12 tablespoons (1½ sticks) unsalted butter, softened

1 cup granulated sugar

2 large egg yolks

1½ cups gluten-free all-purpose flour blend (we've used Arrowhead Mills Gluten Free All Purpose Baking Mix)

1 cup raspberry preserves

6 ounces semisweet chocolate chips

½ cup pecans (about 4 ounces), chopped

½ cup shredded coconut

These versatile little treats just might be the tastiest raspberry bars we've ever tried, and some of the prettiest. Luckily, they are easy to make and can be personalized to suit most any taste. You can top the raspberry layer with chocolate, coconut, nuts, or any combination of those. Below we provide you with the steps to make the super-combo version: just omit or substitute any toppings to suit your own desires!

MAKES 24 TO 30 BARS

STEPS

1 Preheat the oven to 350°F.

2 Grease a 13 × 9–inch baking pan.

3 In a large bowl, beat the butter and sugar until light and fluffy, using a hand-held or stand electric mixer.

4 Add the egg yolks and flour blend and mix until the mixture forms crumbles and starts to stick together.

5 Press the mixture into the prepared baking dish and bake for 20 to 25 minutes, or until the crust is lightly browned.

6 While the crust is baking, place the raspberry preserves in a small bowl and stir for a few minutes, to soften them up and make them more suitable for spreading on the fragile crust.

7 Remove the crust from the oven and let set for 5 minutes.

8 Gently spread the raspberry preserves evenly over the crust. If you accidentally break the crust while spreading the preserves, scoop the preserves off as best as you can and piece the crust back together. The additional baking time will help the crust reset itself.

9 Sprinkle the chocolate chips over the preserves. Place back in the oven for 5 to 10 minutes, or until the chips have melted.

10 Again remove the pan from the oven and use a spatula to spread the melted chocolate out evenly. Before the chocolate cools, sprinkle the nuts and coconut evenly over all. Cool before cutting and serving.

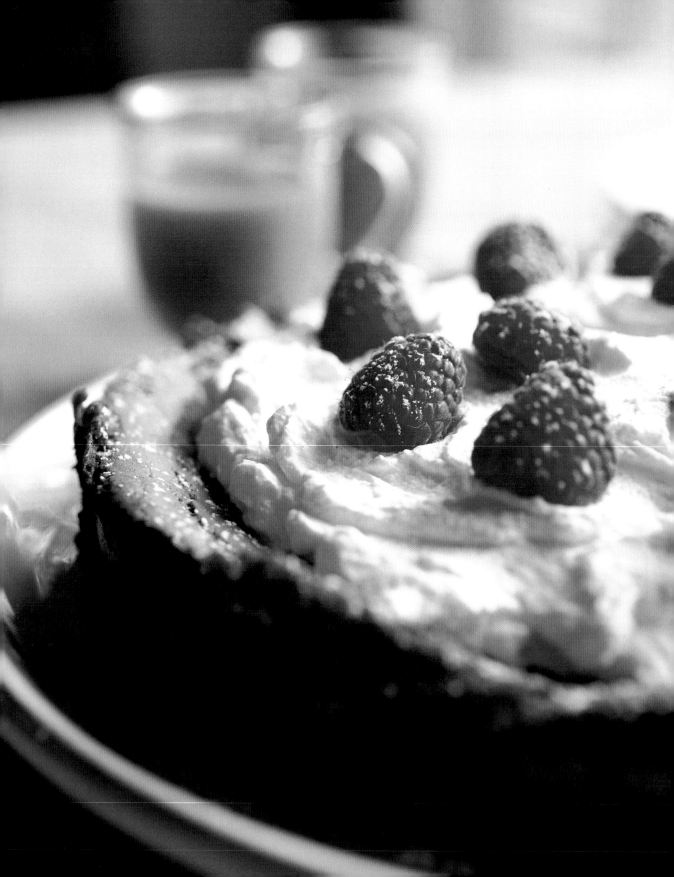

flourless chocolate
and almond cake

INGREDIENTS

4 ounces good-quality dark chocolate with at least 67% cocoa solids, chopped

6 tablespoons (¾ stick) unsalted butter

¾ cup granulated sugar

2 large eggs, lightly whisked

½ teaspoon all-natural vanilla extract

¼ cup plus 2 tablespoons almond meal/flour

½ heaping teaspoon gluten-free baking powder

Freshly whipped cream (optional)

Fresh raspberries (optional)

Confectioner's sugar (powdered sugar) (optional)

This cake is sheer decadence—a rich and chocolate-y cake with a hint of almond running through, a heaping amount of freshly whipped cream, gorgeous raspberries, and just a light dusting of powdered sugar. Wow! This is one indulgence that is completely worth it. Don't be surprised if the center of the cake caves in a bit once cooled—this is perfectly normal. It is easily concealed by the whipped cream and raspberries, so no one will ever notice. Moreover, this cake is so deliriously delicious, no one will care! We suggest making it in a 9-inch springform cake pan, which makes freeing it from the pan much easier. Make sure you use a good-quality dark chocolate or baker's chocolate with at least 67 to 70 percent cocoa solids. Cocoa solids are a blend of cocoa mass and cocoa butter. The higher the percentage, the richer the chocolate and the more beautifully it melts. Green & Black's Baking Bar works wonderfully for this recipe. So it's worth spending a bit extra on a good-quality dark chocolate for this. Yes. You have died and gone into a chocolate-coma heaven!

SERVES 8 TO 10

STEPS

❶ Preheat the oven to 350°F.

❷ Lightly grease a 9-inch springform pan and line the bottom with a piece of parchment paper cut to fit.

❸ Place the chocolate in a heat-proof glass bowl and set the bowl over a small saucepan of simmering water. Once the chocolate is melted, remove the bowl from over the saucepan immediately and set aside.

❹ In a large bowl, cream the butter and sugar together until light and fluffy, using either a hand-held or stand electric mixer.

❺ Add the eggs and vanilla extract and gently beat for 1 minute, until well incorporated.

❻ Slowly and gently fold in the melted chocolate until thoroughly combined.

(recipe continues)

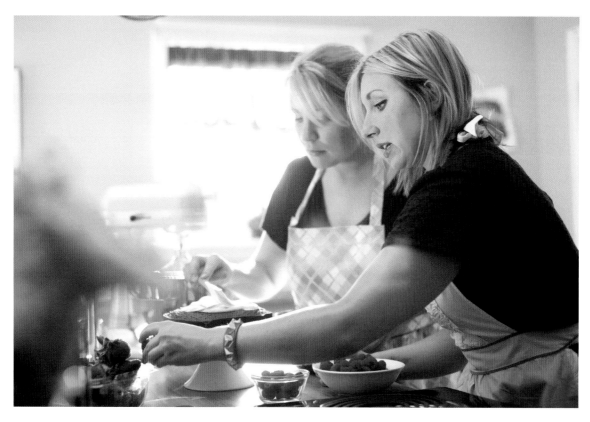

STEPS (CONT.)

7 In a small bowl, stir the almond meal/flour and baking powder to mix well. Add to the chocolate mixture and fold thoroughly together.

8 Pour the batter into the prepared springform pan and bake for 28 to 30 minutes, or until a skewer inserted in the cake comes away clean. The cake should be firm in the middle, not wiggly.

9 Leave to cool in the pan completely. Don't panic if the center of the cake caves in a bit once cooled.

10 Once the cake is fully cooled, release the sides of the springform. Hold a plate over the top of the cake and gently flip it over. Remove the pan bottom to expose the parchment-lined bottom of the cake. Gently peel off the paper.

11 Take another plate or a serving platter, and holding it against the bottom of the cake, flip it all again so the top of the cake is upright. The side of the cake that was facing up in the pan should again be facing up on your plate or serving platter.

12 Place in the refrigerator for 30 minutes to 1 hour to allow the cake to firm up and set.

13 If desired for serving, top with a heaping amount of freshly whipped cream, fresh raspberries, and a dusting of confectioner's sugar.

14 Store the cake in the refrigerator until ready to serve.

peanut butter–cornflake cookies

INGREDIENTS

3¾ cups gluten-free cornflakes

¾ cup granulated sugar

¾ cup light corn syrup

1 cup plus 2 tablespoons peanut butter

Years ago, Jessie's friend Kristy made cookies similar to these. After her diagnosis, Jessie altered the recipe so she could eat them again. These cookies are *very* heavy, so you probably won't need to make more than one recipe's worth if they're just for your family. And a warning: the peanut butter mixture gets very hot, so be careful not to burn yourself while stirring or scooping the cookies. You will find these are a delicious and interesting twist on the usual peanut butter classic. You'll never want a plain old peanut butter cookie again—unless, of course, it's one of our fantastic gluten-free Peanut Butter Cookies from page 193!

MAKES 8 TO 12 LARGE COOKIES

STEPS

❶ Pour the cornflakes into a large bowl and set aside. Cover a baking tray with aluminum foil and set aside.

❷ In a medium-size nonstick saucepan, heat the sugar and corn syrup over medium heat. Stirring almost constantly, cook until the mixture is almost clear, 5 to 10 minutes.

❸ Add the peanut butter and continue stirring until the peanut butter is incorporated and the mixture is of an even consistency.

❹ Carefully pour the hot peanut butter mixture over the cornflakes in the bowl. Use a wooden spoon to stir gently but thoroughly, until all the cornflakes are covered.

❺ Scoop the mixture by heaping spoonfuls onto the foil-covered cookie sheet. Let cool before serving.

pineapple upside-down cake

INGREDIENTS

⅔ cup granulated sugar

½ cup water

2½ cups chopped pineapple pieces (about two 14-ounce cans, drained)

8 tablespoons (1 stick) unsalted butter, softened to room temperature

⅔ cup (packed) soft light brown sugar

2 large eggs

¼ cup full-fat plain Greek yogurt

1 cup gluten-free all-purpose flour blend (we've used Arrowhead Mills Gluten Free All Purpose Baking Mix)

2 heaping teaspoons gluten-free baking powder

1½ teaspoons pumpkin pie spice (blend of cinnamon, nutmeg, ginger, and allspice)

½ teaspoon xanthan gum

½ cup almond meal/flour

This is a gluten-free take on a delicious old favorite. The beauty of this recipe is its versatility. You literally can use any fruit you fancy, especially what is in season. Try it with apples, pears, or bananas in the winter, rhubarb in the spring, or blackberries in the summer. We are giving you room for creative control so you can make this recipe your own. We do *not* advise using a springform pan for this because the syrup will literally go everywhere. Use a 9- or 10-inch cake pan instead, or, for an impressive presentation, make this dish in a clear glass ovenproof or Pyrex dish that you can invert. People will bow to you and your cake-making skills.

SERVES 8

STEPS

❶ Preheat the oven to 350°F. Grease a 9- or 10-inch cake pan, making sure all sides are well covered.

❷ Line the bottom with a piece of parchment paper cut to fit.

❸ In a small nonstick saucepan, stir the granulated sugar and ¼ cup of the water over low heat until the sugar is dissolved, about 3 to 4 minutes.

❹ Once the sugar is dissolved, turn the heat to medium high and boil, without stirring, until the mixture has a golden, toffee color, about 13 to 15 minutes. After the mixture has been caramelizing for about 10 minutes, quickly bring the remaining ¼ cup water to a boil in either a kettle or saucepan.

❺ Once the toffee syrup has caramelized and achieved its toffee color, turn off the heat and quickly move the pan into the sink.

❻ Very carefully add the boiling water to the pan and stand back. Make sure you are wearing long sleeves or oven mitts when doing this! The mixture will bubble up and sizzle into the consistency of a thick syrup in 1 to 2 minutes. This is your toffee syrup topping.

❼ Once the mixture has stopped bubbling loudly, very quickly stir to blend, and then pour the syrup immediately over the bottom of the prepared cake pan. You must do this with speed before the syrup gets too thick to work with.

8 Pour the pineapple or fruit of choice on top of the syrup in an even layer and set the pan aside.

9 In a large bowl, cream the butter and brown sugar until soft and fluffy, using either a hand-held or stand electric mixer.

10 Add the eggs, one at a time, while beating continuously.

11 Fold in the Greek yogurt and gently mix until well combined.

12 In another bowl sift together the flour blend, baking powder, pumpkin pie spice, and xanthan gum. Add the almond meal/flour and stir to mix well.

13 Add the dry ingredients to the butter mixture and fold thoroughly together.

14 Spoon the batter over the pineapple and syrup, spreading it out evenly as you go.

15 Bake for 45 minutes, or until a toothpick inserted in the cake comes away clean.

16 Let cool in the pan fully, before carefully inverting the cake onto a serving dish or plate.

17 Gently peel off the parchment paper and discard before serving. Store the cake in the refrigerator until ready to serve.

lemon *and* poppy seed syrup cake

INGREDIENTS

8 tablespoons (1 stick) unsalted butter, softened to room temperature

1 cup granulated sugar

¾ cup almond meal/flour

½ teaspoon all-natural vanilla extract

2 large eggs

⅓ cup lemon juice (from roughly 2 lemons)

Scant 2 tablespoons finely grated lemon zest (from roughly 2 lemons)

⅓ cup finely ground cornmeal or polenta flour

1½ teaspoons poppy seeds

½ teaspoon gluten-free baking powder

1 tablespoon cornstarch

2 tablespoons water

We love to have this cake on standby in case friends or family drop in for a cup of tea or coffee and a chat. It's surprisingly easy to put together and always goes down well, celiac disease or not. We seem to always forget to leave our butter out to soften, so you can cheat by microwaving it quickly for 30 seconds or so if needed. You can also make this cake in a loaf pan instead. Jilly particularly likes the silicone versions out there that make inverting the cake for glazing exceptionally easy. Just allow your cake to cool fully before attempting the "invert the cake with 2 plates" magic trick . . . we speak from the experience of personal disasters (though the dog seems to love that mishap!). Patience really is a virtue. If using a loaf pan instead of an 8- or 9-inch cake pan, you may need to adjust your baking time to 45 to 50 minutes.

SERVES 6 TO 8

STEPS

❶ Preheat the oven to 350°F.

❷ Grease the bottom and sides of an 8- or 9-inch cake pan or loaf pan. Line the bottom with a piece of parchment paper cut to fit.

❸ In a large bowl, cream the butter and ¾ cup of the sugar until light and fluffy, using either a hand-held or stand electric mixer.

❹ Add the almond meal/flour, vanilla extract, and eggs and beat well to mix thoroughly.

❺ Add 2½ tablespoons of the lemon juice, all but 1 teaspoon of the zest, the cornmeal, poppy seeds, and baking powder, and mix well.

❻ Spoon the batter into the prepared cake pan or loaf pan and spread out evenly. Bake for 30 minutes, or until the top is golden brown and a toothpick inserted comes away clean.

❼ Allow the cake to cool fully, in the pan, before glazing.

❽ While it is cooling, in a small bowl stir the cornstarch and water to blend. Set aside.

❾ When the cake has cooled, make the syrup. In a small non-stick saucepan, whisk together the remaining lemon juice and zest, the remaining sugar, and the cornstarch-water mixture.

10 Set over medium-low heat and bring to a bubble to allow the sauce to thicken, whisking constantly. Once it turns into a thick glaze, turn off the heat and set aside.

11 Invert the cooled cake by holding a plate over the top of the pan and gently flipping it all over to turn the cake out, so the parchment-lined bottom is exposed. Gently peel off the parchment paper and discard.

12 Hold another plate or serving platter against the cake bottom and carefully flip all again so the top of the cake is once again upright.

13 Using a small spatula, glaze the entire cake, top and sides, with the lemon-syrup glaze.

14 Place in the refrigerator for 10 minutes to set before cutting and serving.

lemon *and* blackberry cheesecake

INGREDIENTS

2½ cups gluten-free cookies, ginger if possible

4 tablespoons (½ stick) unsalted butter, melted

2 packages (8 ounces each) full-fat cream cheese, softened to room temperature

¾ cup granulated sugar

½ cup crème fraîche or full-fat sour cream

3 large eggs

3 tablespoons lemon juice

1 heaping tablespoon cornstarch dissolved in 2 tablespoons water

1½ teaspoons finely grated lemon zest (roughly zest of 1 lemon)

½ teaspoon all-natural vanilla extract

1 cup fresh blackberries, washed and patted dry

Without question, cheesecake is one of the most luscious desserts on the planet. Everyone loves a good cheesecake, and they will certainly love this one. We find it sets best overnight, but if you can't wait that long before diving in, 6 hours will do. You can substitute blueberries for the blackberries if you prefer, but the beautiful color of the blackberries makes this dish as gorgeous to look at as it is to eat. Blackberries are at their best in the early fall season, when they are at their juiciest but aren't too full of seeds. We suggest using a 9-inch springform pan, which makes the cheesecake's release oh so easy. Everyone who has tasted this cheesecake has asked us for the recipe. Fact is, it's just that dreamy!

SERVES 8 TO 10

STEPS

❶ Lightly grease the bottom and sides of a 9-inch springform pan.

❷ Roughly break up the cookies and place in the bowl of a food processor along with the melted butter. Pulse until the mixture forms crumbs.

❸ Using your fingers, firmly press this mixture, as evenly as possible, over the bottom of the prepared pan to form a crust. Place in the refrigerator to set for 30 minutes.

❹ Preheat the oven to 325°F.

❺ Combine the remaining ingredients except for the blackberries in a large bowl, and using a hand-held or stand electric mixer, beat until blended and smooth.

❻ Remove the pan from the refrigerator and pour the filling mixture over the crust.

❼ Scatter the blackberries over the top of the filling any way you'd like.

❽ Bake for 45 to 50 minutes, until the sides are firm and set but still slightly wiggly in the center.

(recipe continues)

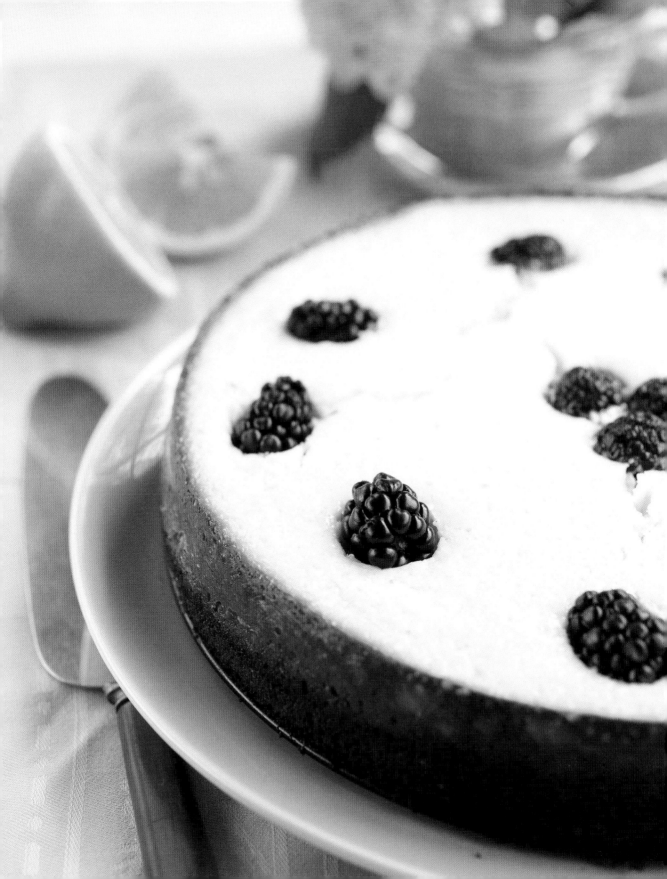

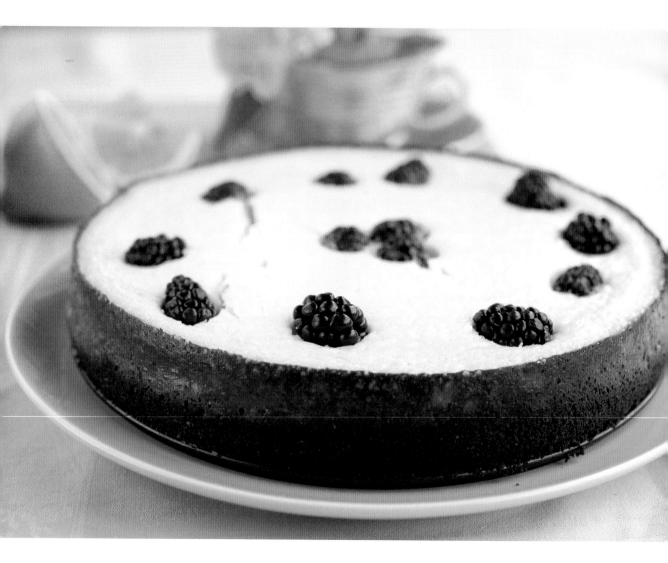

STEPS (CONT.)

9 Cool the cake on a rack or cutting board until it is fully cooled before covering tightly with cling film and placing in the refrigerator for at least 6 hours.

10 When ready to slice and serve, run a sharp knife under warm water briefly and then dry. Run the knife around the inside of the springform and carefully release the sides.

11 Again carefully, place the cake on a serving dish and use the same knife-preparation technique to slice the cake. With the warm knife, you'll be able to cut perfect slices with ease while maintaining the cake's integrity.

peanut butter cookies

INGREDIENTS

1 cup creamy peanut butter

½ cup sugar

½ cup light brown sugar

1 large egg, beaten

1 teaspoon vanilla extract

Boy, how we love peanut butter—peanut butter on gluten-free toast, peanut butter with apples, and, of course, peanut butter cookies. Jessie's son, Jude, loves peanut butter so much he eats it all by itself right out of the jar! These amazingly tasty little peanut butter cookies are so easy to make but they are so, so delicious. This is a perfect recipe for little ones to assist in making. They love stirring everything together, using the fork to press the cookies down, and—naturally—eating them warm straight out of the oven.

MAKES 24 COOKIES

STEPS

❶ Preheat the oven to 350°F and make sure the oven rack is in the center position.

❷ Combine all the ingredients in a bowl and stir well with a wooden spoon until smooth.

❸ Divide the dough into 24 portions, about 1 heaping tablespoon each. Roll each portion between your hands to form a smooth ball.

❹ Place the balls of dough on ungreased cookie sheets, leaving 1 inch of space between them. Press down with a fork in two directions to form a cross-hatch pattern. You should get 12 cookies per sheet.

❺ Bake one sheet at a time in the oven until the cookies are risen and lightly golden, about 10 minutes.

❻ Remove the cookies from the oven and let cool before removing them from the baking sheet with a metal spatula.

❼ Repeat with the remaining sheet of cookies.

new orleans–style pecan pie
with gluten-free crust

Recipe courtesy Emeril Lagasse, copyright MSLO, Inc., all rights reserved.

INGREDIENTS

filling

- 1 cup light Karo syrup
- 3 whole eggs plus 1 yolk, beaten
- ½ cup light brown sugar
- ½ cup white sugar
- 2 tablespoons melted butter
- 1 teaspoon vanilla extract
- ¼ teaspoon almond extract
- 1½ cups shelled pecan halves or pieces
- 1 gluten-free pie crust, partially blind baked as described in recipe below

Pecan pie is a New Orleans institution and most certainly a Lagasse one, too. We make this pie several times throughout the year—Mardi Gras, Thanksgiving, and Christmas at least! It's just heaven in a bite. Jilly likes to sprinkle a few chocolate chips on top of hers before baking for an even more decadent pie. Light Karo syrup is simply light corn syrup and should be readily available at your local grocery store, in the baking section. Dad's delicious gluten-free pie crust recipe yields 2 pie crusts, so feel free to freeze one until you need it. You can use it for savory or sweet dishes, so get creative and let us know what you come up with! Everyone loves a blank canvas, don't they? Slice a lil' New Orleans lovin' with this delicious pie and enjoy!

SERVES 8 TO 10

STEPS

filling

1 Preheat the oven to 350°F.

2 In a bowl, combine all of the ingredients except for the pecans and the pie crust. Mix well.

3 Arrange the pecans on the bottom of the partially blind baked pie crust (instructions on page 196) and carefully pour the filling over them. The pecans will float to the top.

4 Bake for 55 to 60 minutes, or until the filling has set and reaches an internal temperature of 200°F.

5 Allow the pie to cool on a rack for at least two hours before serving.

(recipe continues)

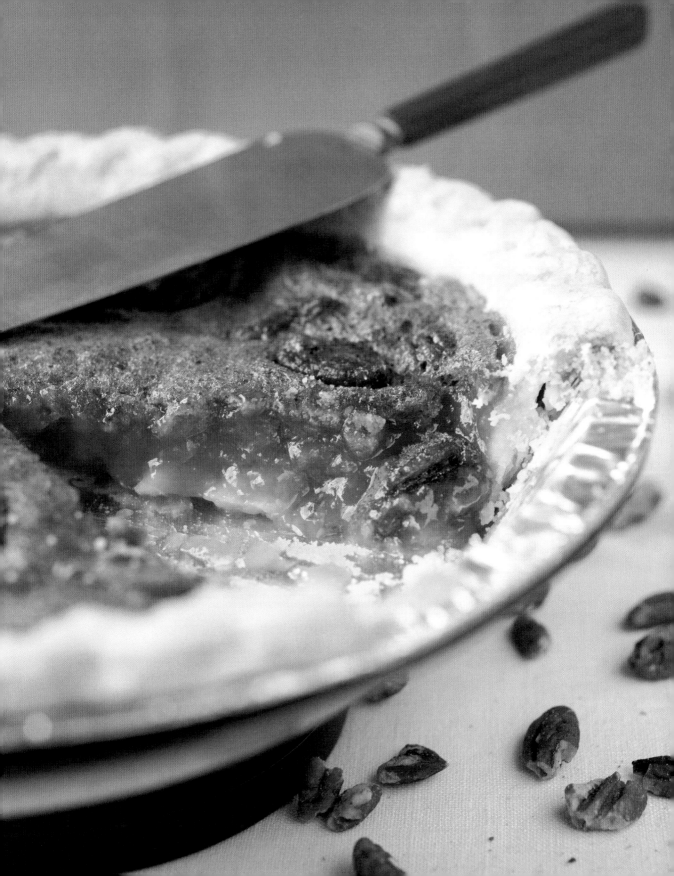

INGREDIENTS (CONT.)

crust

1 cup white rice flour

¾ cup tapioca flour

¾ cup potato starch

1 heaping teaspoon xanthan gum

¾ teaspoon salt

1 tablespoon plus 1 teaspoon sugar

½ cup shortening

¼ cup butter

1 egg, lightly beaten

1 tablespoon vinegar

2 to 3 tablespoons ice water

Sweet rice flour for dusting

STEPS (CONT.)

crust

❶ Preheat the oven to 450°F.

❷ In a medium bowl, whisk together the rice and tapioca flours, potato starch, xanthan gum, salt, and sugar.

❸ Cut in the shortening and butter.

❹ Blend together the beaten egg, vinegar, and cold water in a separate bowl.

❺ Stir into the flour mixture and knead into a ball. You cannot overknead this dough.

❻ Form dough into two balls and place in a bowl; cover and refrigerate for 30 minutes.

❼ Remove and roll out one ball of the dough between two sheets of parchment paper dusted with sweet rice flour. Remove the top sheet of parchment and invert the dough and drop it into the pan. The dough is delicate and should be handled with care. Shape the dough around the edges if necessary, using any extra bits and pasting with a little extra cool water, as you would with normal pie dough.

❽ Repeat this process with the second ball of dough to form a second pie crust.

❾ Line the crusts with parchment, fill with pie weights, and bake for 10 to 12 minutes, or until the dough is lightly golden around the top edges and the bottom of the pie pastry is opaque and dry.

❿ Freeze the second crust for another use. Allow the crust to cool before making the filling.

note: *The dough does not hold well, so we advise either making 2 pies or partially blind baking as described above and freezing for a later date.*

peach crumble *in* grand marnier *and* cinnamon custard

INGREDIENTS

5 cups sliced peaches (about 4 to 5 small fresh peaches, pitted and peeled, or 24 ounces frozen peaches, thawed)

2½ cups gluten-free cookies, ginger if possible

2½ tablespoons unsalted butter, melted

⅓ cup Marshmallow Fluff topping

1¼ teaspoons ground cinnamon

1 can (15 ounces) ambrosia custard

3½ teaspoons Grand Marnier liqueur

Vanilla ice cream, for serving (optional)

This is a gorgeous dessert that is quick and easy to assemble and makes a perfect summer dish when peaches are in season. They are at their juiciest from June to late August. You can use either pink or white-fleshed peaches for this dish. If fresh peaches aren't an option, you can substitute all-natural frozen peaches. We suggest avoiding a canned variety, as they are far too sugary. For this dish we use canned ambrosia custard, which you should be able to find in your local grocery or specialty store, in the British section. We found ours at the local World Market. Serve this crumble warm, preferably with a nice scoop of your favorite vanilla ice cream.

SERVES 6 TO 8

STEPS

1 Preheat the oven to 350°F.

2 Place the peaches in a large bowl and set aside.

3 In the bowl of a food processor, combine the cookies and melted butter and pulse a few times until big crumbs form.

4 Transfer the crumbs to a medium-size bowl and add the marshmallow topping and 1 teaspoon of the cinnamon. Using a fork or your hands, work until well combined and the mixture resembles crumbles. Set aside.

5 In another bowl, whisk together the custard, Grand Marnier, and remaining ¼ teaspoon cinnamon until mixed.

6 Pour this mixture over the sliced peaches in their bowl and gently mix.

7 Pour the peach mixture into an ungreased 11½ × 8-inch baking dish.

8 Using your fingers, crumble the topping over the peach mixture, making sure to cover completely.

9 Bake for 25 minutes, or until bubbling around the edges. Serve immediately, with scoops of vanilla ice cream, if desired.

mrs. gloria's fruit pizza

Jessie's friend Marcus became one of this book's loyal test subjects, sampling everything we turned out. Marcus's mom, Mrs. Gloria, served up this great fruit pizza for Marcus's thirtieth birthday party, and in honor of him, this is Jessie's take on Mrs. Gloria's original. Although we prefer to make one large, 12-inch pizza, you can also use a 3.5-inch, round cookie cutter to make individual mini pizzas. Any kind of ripe fruit will work on this pizza, though here we've used peaches, strawberries, and grapes. Also, it's best to make this pizza—big or small version—a day in advance, so the sugar cookie crust has a chance to soften with the toppings a little.

SERVES 12 TO 16 OR MAKES 10 TO 12 MINI PIZZAS

INGREDIENTS

crust

Cooking spray or oil

2 cups gluten-free all-purpose flour blend (we've used Arrowhead Mills Gluten Free All Purpose Baking Mix)

¼ teaspoon salt

½ teaspoon gluten-free baking powder

8 ounces (2 sticks) unsalted butter, softened

1 cup granulated sugar

1 tablespoon (packed) light brown sugar

1 large egg

2 teaspoons all-natural vanilla extract

topping

1 package (8 ounces) cream cheese, softened

⅓ cup plus 4 teaspoons granulated sugar

Sliced peaches

Sliced strawberries

Sliced grapes

1 cup orange juice

4 teaspoons cornstarch

STEPS

crust

❶ Preheat the oven to 375°F.

❷ Using cooking spray or oil, grease a 12-inch pizza pan or, if making mini pizzas, a large cookie sheet (approximately 17 × 13 inches). In a medium-size bowl, whisk together the flour blend, salt, and baking powder to mix well. Set aside.

❸ In a large bowl, cream the butter, granulated sugar, and light brown sugar until light and fluffy, using a hand-held or stand electric mixer.

❹ Add the egg and vanilla and beat at medium speed until thoroughly incorporated.

❺ On low speed, blend in the dry ingredients and beat until all ingredients are combined.

❻ Spoon the cookie dough onto the prepared pizza pan or cookie sheet, using a spatula to spread it evenly. The dough will be somewhat loose, so it's best to try to spread it rather than roll it.

❼ Bake the dough until the top is an even, light golden brown. This usually takes between 15 to 20 minutes, depending on your oven.

❽ Remove from the oven and let the crust cool completely before adding the topping. If making mini pizzas, wait for the crust to cool before cutting out the circles. Then proceed with the topping steps.

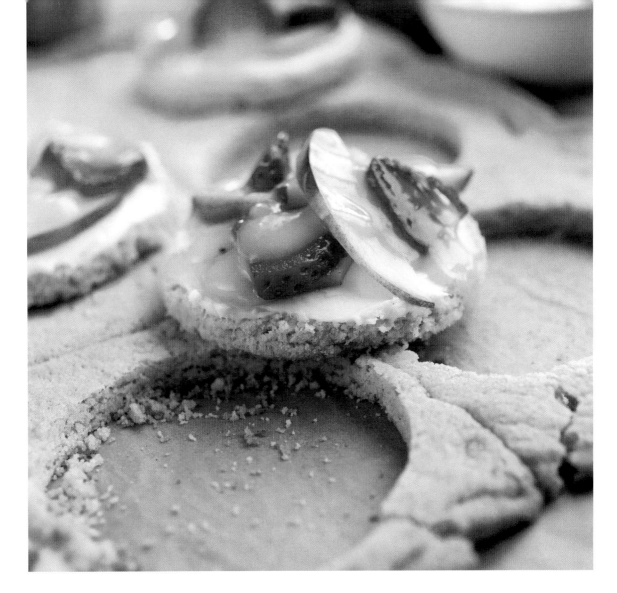

topping

1 In a medium-size bowl, beat the cream cheese and ⅓ cup of the granulated sugar until blended and smooth, using a hand-held or stand electric mixer at medium speed.

2 Spread the cream cheese mixture over the cooled cookie crust in a thin layer.

3 The next step is to add your selection of fruit toppings. You can use as little or as much fruit as desired. We prefer to make an even layer of toppings and not have any fruit overlap any other fruit. But it's up to you.

4 Once the fruit is added, it's time to add the glaze. Whisk the orange juice, remaining 4 teaspoons sugar, and the cornstarch together in a small saucepan. Heat over medium heat, whisking frequently, until the glaze begins to thicken.

5 Remove the pan from the heat, and using a small ladle or spoon, spoon the glaze evenly over the fruit topping.

6 Chill the pizza for at least 30 minutes and up to 24 hours, and then slice and serve.

apple betty

INGREDIENTS

4 cups sliced Granny Smith apples (2 to 3 apples, peeled and cored)

2 tablespoons orange juice

3 tablespoons (packed) light brown sugar

¼ cup plus 2 tablespoons gluten-free all-purpose flour blend (we've used Arrowhead Mills Gluten Free All Purpose Baking Mix)

½ cup granulated sugar

½ teaspoon ground cinnamon

Pinch of ground nutmeg

4 tablespoons (½ stick) unsalted butter, softened

Vanilla ice cream, for serving (optional)

When Jessie evacuated New Orleans after Hurricane Katrina, she spent three months living in a Homewood Suites Hotel in Virginia. Having only a toaster oven forced her to get creative in preparing her favorite foods. This recipe is a terrific replacement for a full-size apple pie and is absolutely delicious served with a scoop of vanilla ice cream. Plus, you can even cook it in the toaster oven!

SERVES 6 TO 8

STEPS

❶ Preheat the oven to 375°F.

❷ In a medium-size bowl, toss the apples with the orange juice and 1 tablespoon of the brown sugar to coat well.

❸ Pour the apple mixture into an ungreased 9-inch deep-dish pie plate and set aside.

❹ In another bowl, combine the flour blend, granulated sugar, remaining 2 tablespoons brown sugar, cinnamon, and nutmeg. Using a fork, cut in the softened butter, creating crumbly clumps.

❺ Once all the flour mixture is incorporated into crumbles, gently spoon the crumbles on top of the apples in the pie plate. Try to spread the mixture evenly over the entire surface.

❻ Bake for 40 to 50 minutes, or until the apples are fork tender and the crumbles are browned.

❼ Serve warm, with vanilla ice cream, if desired.

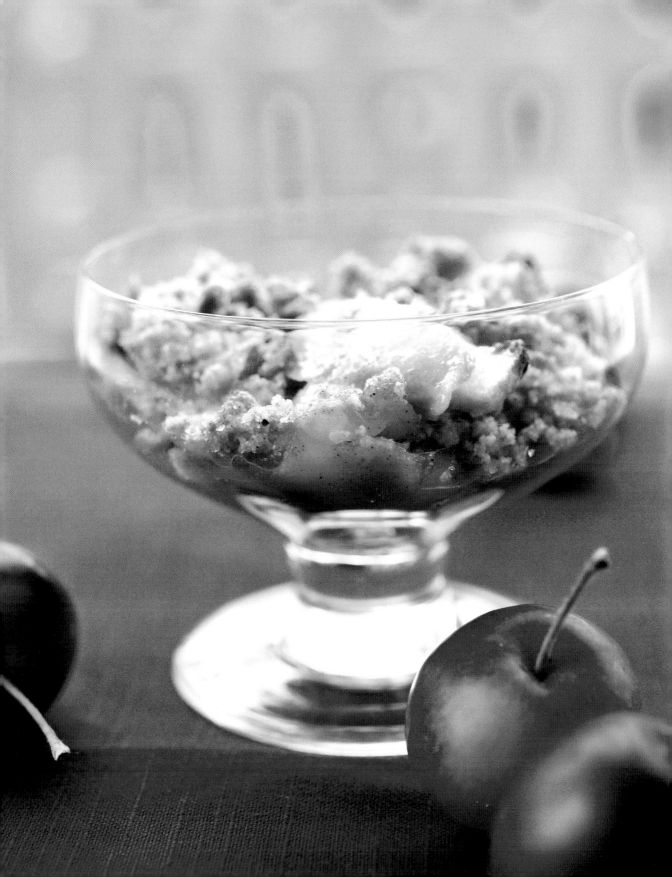

lemon curd custards

INGREDIENTS

4 large eggs

⅔ cup granulated sugar

½ teaspoon all-natural vanilla extract

⅓ cup lemon juice (from roughly 2 large lemons)

3 tablespoons finely grated lemon zest (from roughly 2 large lemons)

½ cup heavy cream

Strawberries or whipped cream, for garnish (optional)

Jilly's love of lemon curd inspired this sweet and creamy dish. Lemon curd is a British staple, and despite the name, it is not a curd at all! It is actually a very rich dessert spread made of lemons, sugar, eggs, and butter. Very naughty indeed! Traditionally, it would be served with scones or bread at afternoon tea or used as a dessert filling for cakes, tarts, and pastries. It's the sweet counterpart to a good hot sauce—you can put it on just about anything and it'll taste great! Use the freshest lemons and eggs possible, as it will help with the vibrancy in color and flavor. You can place a few dark chocolate chips into the center of the custards right before baking for an extra surprise. This will make four 8-ounce ramekins' worth of custard. If you like lemons, you are going to love this treat!

MAKES 4 CUSTARDS

STEPS

❶ Preheat the oven to 325°F. Have ready four 8-ounce oven-proof ramekins.

❷ Prepare a water bath in a deep oven-proof baking dish, such as a Pyrex dish or a small roasting pan, by filling it halfway with cold water.

❸ In a medium-size bowl, whisk together the eggs, sugar, and vanilla until thick.

❹ Stir in the lemon juice and zest, and whisk well.

❺ Add in the cream and stir gently, so all ingredients are well mixed.

❻ Pour the mixture into the ramekins, trying to distribute it evenly. Place the ramekins in the baking dish.

❼ Bake for 30 to 40 minutes. You want the centers of the custards to be set before removing them from the oven, though they will still be wiggly.

❽ Carefully remove the custards from the water bath and allow them to cool fully on a heat-resistant surface, such as a cutting board.

❾ Once fully cooled, cover each custard tightly with cling film and refrigerate until needed.

❿ Serve with a small dollop of whipped cream or a few strawberries on top, if desired.

lemon squares

INGREDIENTS

1 cup plus 2 tablespoons gluten-free all-purpose flour blend (we've used Arrowhead Mills Gluten Free All Purpose Baking Mix)

¼ cup confectioner's sugar (powdered sugar), plus additional for garnish

3 large eggs

6 tablespoons (¾ stick) butter, softened

3 tablespoons lemon juice

1 cup granulated sugar

¼ teaspoon gluten-free baking powder

One of Jessie's favorite treats has always been lemon squares. The bakery up the street from her house knows her by name because she used to go in looking for fresh lemon squares so frequently. It was only natural that after her diagnosis, she'd have to create her own gluten-free version. And this is it. The acidity of the lemon is balanced perfectly by the sweetness of the sugar. These squares are a little more crumbly than traditional lemon squares, but they stay together just fine.

MAKES 12 TO 16 SQUARES

STEPS

❶ Preheat the oven to 350°F.

❷ Grease an 8 × 8–inch baking dish.

❸ Mix 1 cup of the flour blend with the confectioner's sugar. Lightly beat 1 of the eggs. Using a fork or wooden spoon, mix in the butter and the beaten egg until the mixture forms crumbles and begins to stick together.

❹ Press the mixture into the prepared baking dish and bake for 20 to 25 minutes, or until light golden brown.

❺ Right before you remove the crust from the oven, usually at about the 20-minute mark, beat the lemon juice, remaining 2 eggs, and granulated sugar in a small bowl until thoroughly incorporated.

❻ In a small bowl, stir the remaining 2 tablespoons flour blend with the baking powder to mix well. Add this mixture to the lemon juice mixture and whisk gently but thoroughly to blend.

❼ Remove the crust from the oven and immediately pour on the lemon mixture. Remember, your baking dish is hot! Return the dish to the oven for another 20 to 25 minutes, or until the filling is set.

❽ Remove from the oven, sprinkle with additional confectioner's sugar, and let cool before cutting into squares.

grandma cabral's banana nut bread

INGREDIENTS

8 tablespoons (1 stick) unsalted butter

1 cup (packed) light brown sugar

½ teaspoon all-natural vanilla extract

2 large eggs

3 large (or 4 small) very ripe bananas

⅓ cup applesauce

Pinch of ground cinnamon

1 cup gluten-free all-purpose flour blend (we've used Arrowhead Mills Gluten Free All Purpose Baking Mix)

¼ cup cornstarch

2 teaspoons gluten-free baking powder

2 teaspoons salt

½ cup walnuts, roughly chopped

Growing up, we both knew it was a very special treat to visit our great-grandmother Cabral. If we close our eyes, we can still remember all the wonderful smells that poured out of her house—a mixture of her Portuguese soup, chourico, and, of course, her famous banana bread. Every time we would leave, she'd send us home with a loaf of our very own to take with us, always wrapped in aluminum foil. The excitement we got out of opening that crunchy foil once we were home was grander than opening up a bar of Willy Wonka's chocolate containing that winning golden ticket! During our visit, Grandma would be in the kitchen cooking while we played with our cousins or just sat and watched her every move. It is one of our earliest memories of the happiness food, when made with love, can bring to those around you.

Grandma Cabral never wrote down her recipes; she just cooked with her heart. It took Jilly a while to replicate this dish, but we think we've cracked it. The key is using bananas that are almost bad! The browner the better, as they are a bit sweeter that way. The applesauce keeps this bread nice and moist. We hope it makes your house smell as enticing as we remember Grandma Cabral's house smelling. Bake some banana nut bread and make some memories!

MAKES ONE 9 x 5 x 3–INCH LOAF

STEPS

❶ Preheat the oven to 350°F. Grease a 9 x 5 x 3–inch loaf pan.

❷ In a medium-size bowl, cream the butter, sugar, and vanilla extract until light and fluffy, using either a hand-held or stand electric mixer.

❸ Add the eggs and beat again until well mixed.

❹ In a separate bowl, mash the bananas, applesauce, and cinnamon together using a fork or potato masher.

❺ Stir the banana mixture into the butter mixture to mix well.

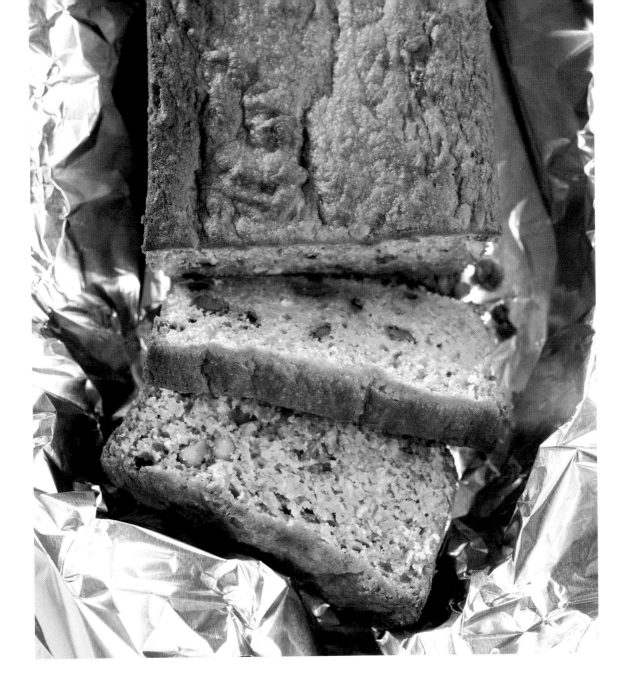

6 In another bowl, sift together the flour blend, cornstarch, baking powder, and salt.

7 Slowly add the dry ingredients, in batches, to the banana mixture, beating well to mix. Fold in the walnut pieces and pour the batter into the prepared loaf pan.

8 Bake for 1¼ to 1½ hours, until the top is golden brown and a toothpick inserted in the middle of the bread comes away clean.

9 Serve warm.

summer fruit crèmes brûlées

INGREDIENTS

1½ cups fruit of choice
(we've used a mix
of strawberries and
nectarines)

1½ teaspoons water

2 large eggs plus 2 large yolks

4 tablespoons granulated
sugar

1 cup (8 ounces) heavy cream

Seeds from 1 vanilla bean
pod split lengthwise and
scraped out

People are always impressed by these gorgeous crèmes brûlées, whether you have a blowtorch to complete the final presentation or not. You can use any mix of fresh fruit you like; peaches, raspberries, and strawberries all work fantastically well. The freshly scraped vanilla beans make a wonderful addition to the creamy filling. If you do have a mini crème brûlée blowtorch, you can brown and crisp the sugar-coated tops tableside for your guests. This extra bit of showmanship will put you at the top of everyone's must-invite list!

MAKES 4 CRÈMES BRÛLÉES

STEPS

1 Preheat the oven to 325°F and have ready four 8-ounce oven-proof ramekins.

2 In a small saucepan over medium-high heat, bring the fruit and the water to a bubbly, gentle boil, and then turn the heat to low and let simmer until the fruit has softened, about 3 to 4 minutes, stirring frequently.

3 Turn off the heat and let the fruit cool in the pan.

4 In a medium-size bowl, whisk together the eggs and egg yolks and 2 tablespoons of the sugar until light and frothy. Set aside.

5 In another small nonstick saucepan, gently warm together the cream and vanilla bean seeds over low heat, stirring often for 2 to 3 minutes.

6 Turn the heat to medium and bring the cream to a gentle boil, stirring frequently so it doesn't stick to the bottom of the pan.

7 As soon as the cream comes to a boil, quickly take it off the heat and slowly pour it into the egg mixture, whisking continuously. Take your time with this step, as you want to temper the mixture, and if you pour the warm cream in too quickly, you could break the mixture or curdle the eggs.

8 Whisk well, and then transfer to a large jug or measuring cup and set aside.

9 Bring water to a boil in a kettle or saucepan.

10 Using a slotted spoon, divide the fruit compote evenly among the ramekins, using only the fruit and discarding any remaining juices.

11 Pour the custard mixture over the fruit, distributing it evenly among the ramekins.

12 Place the ramekins in a deep-sided baking dish set on an oven rack.

13 Carefully pour the boiling water into the dish making sure it comes only halfway up the sides of the ramekins. Be very careful not to get any water in the ramekins.

14 Bake for 25 to 30 minutes, or until the custards are firmly set and not wiggly.

15 Carefully take the ramekins out of the water-filled dish and let cool on a heat-resistant surface, such as a cutting board.

16 Once fully cooled, wrap each custard tightly with cling film and refrigerate for at least 1 hour or up to 24.

17 Before serving, sprinkle with the remaining 2 tablespoons sugar, divided among the 4 ramekins.

18 Caramelize the tops by either using a mini blowtorch or putting them under a very hot broiler until just brown and bubbly, about 2 minutes. Serve immediately.

pumpkin spice muffins

INGREDIENTS

½ cup peeled, seeded, and cubed pumpkin or yellow squash (about 4 ounces) or ½ cup canned pumpkin

1¼ cups gluten-free all-purpose flour blend (we've used Arrowhead Mills Gluten Free All Purpose Baking Mix)

½ cup (packed) light brown sugar

2 teaspoons gluten-free baking powder

1 heaping teaspoon pumpkin pie spice (mix of cinnamon, ginger, nutmeg, and cloves)

Pinch of nutmeg

⅓ cup dried natural cranberries

½ cup milk, any % fat you prefer

1 large egg

½ cup orange juice, pulp-free

2½ tablespoons grated orange zest (from roughly 1 orange)

½ stick (4 tablespoons) unsalted butter, melted

½ teaspoon all-natural vanilla extract

These muffins scream that fall has arrived! They are quick to make and perfect to eat on a chilly autumn morning, perhaps reading by a warm, cozy fire. They are also a delightful way to use up any pumpkin flesh you're stuck with after Halloween. You can substitute an equal amount of canned pumpkin as well, if it makes things easier. The orange zest adds a nice warmth to these muffins, subtle yet perfectly savory. Bake off a batch and go impress your neighbors.

MAKES 12 MUFFINS

STEPS

1 If using canned pumpkin, place in a large bowl and skip to step 4. In a medium-size saucepan, pour water over the pumpkin flesh with just enough water to cover it.

2 On medium heat, cook the pumpkin until fork tender, about 10 to 15 minutes.

3 Strain the pumpkin and place in a large bowl. With a potato masher, mash the pumpkin to a smooth consistency. Set aside and let cool.

4 Preheat the oven to 400°F.

5 Line one 12-cup muffin tin or two 6-cup tins with paper muffin cups.

6 In a medium-size bowl, combine the flour blend, sugar, baking powder, pumpkin pie spice, nutmeg, and cranberries and stir with a fork to mix well.

7 In a separate bowl, combine the milk, egg, orange juice and zest, butter, and vanilla extract. Stir well to blend thoroughly.

8 Add the cooled pumpkin flesh (or canned pumpkin) to the wet mixture and stir well.

9 Gently but thoroughly fold the dry ingredients into the pumpkin mixture. It's okay if the batter still contains a few lumps.

10 Spoon the batter into the 12 muffin cups, dividing evenly, and bake for 20 to 25 minutes,

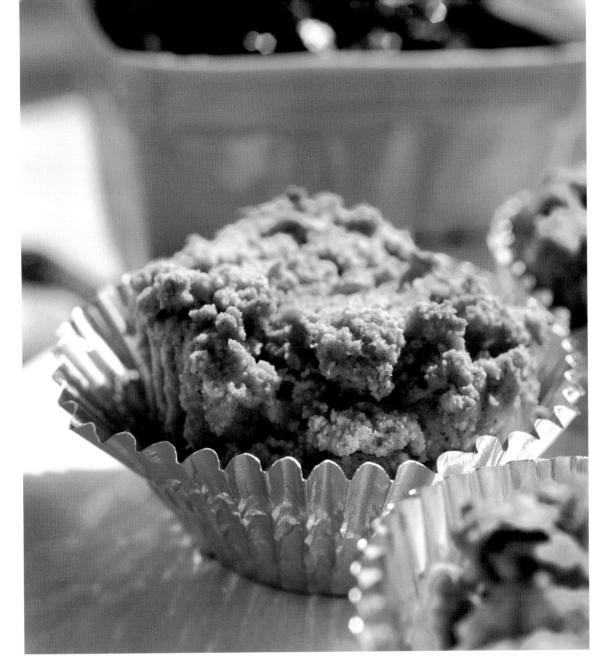

or until a toothpick inserted in the center comes out clean. The muffins will still be moist, and they won't "rise" like conventional muffins, so don't be worried if they collapse or cave in a bit in the center. Perfectly normal.

11 Allow the muffins to cool to room temperature in the tins before placing in the refrigerator for 30 minutes to set.

12 After 30 minutes, take out and serve.

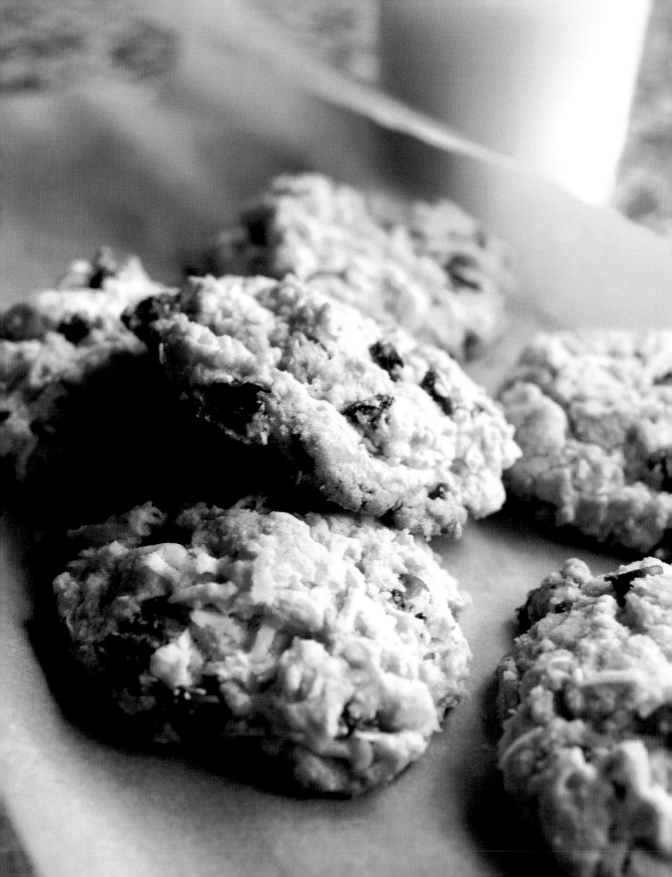

coconut chocolate-chip cookies

INGREDIENTS

2 cups gluten-free all-purpose flour blend (we've used Arrowhead Mills Gluten Free All Purpose Baking Mix)

½ teaspoon gluten-free baking powder

½ teaspoon salt

12 tablespoons (1½ sticks) unsalted butter, softened

1 cup (packed) light brown sugar

½ cup granulated sugar

1 large egg plus 1 large yolk

2 teaspoons all-natural vanilla extract

½ to ¾ cup semisweet chocolate chips

2½ cups sweetened flaked coconut

Cookies were one of the things Jessie missed the most when she was first diagnosed. However, these cookies taste so good you'll never miss the gluten! This recipe produces cookies somewhat reminiscent of that Girl Scout cookie favorite, the Samoa, though these cookies are crunchy rather than super chewy. You can also eliminate the coconut for a terrific traditional chocolate-chip cookie. Try serving them warm, with vanilla ice cream for a delicious cookie à la mode!

MAKES 12 TO 18 COOKIES, DEPENDING ON SIZE

STEPS

❶ Preheat the oven to 325°F.

❷ Grease 2 large baking trays.

❸ In a medium-size bowl, whisk together the flour blend, baking powder, and salt. Set aside.

❹ In a large bowl, cream together the butter and sugars until light and fluffy, using a hand-held or stand electric mixer on medium speed.

❺ Add the egg, egg yolk, and vanilla and beat thoroughly until blended.

❻ Reducing the mixer speed to low, gradually add the flour mixture and beat until just combined.

❼ Stir in the chocolate chips and the coconut until just incorporated.

❽ Spoon the dough in approximately ¼-cup balls onto the prepared baking trays, leaving about 2 inches between the balls.

❾ Bake until the cookies are a light golden brown. The edges will be crispy, while the centers will be soft and almost uncooked looking. This can take anywhere from 15 to 20 minutes, depending on your oven.

❿ Remove from the oven and let the cookies cool on the sheets.

white chocolate
and cherry butter cookies

INGREDIENTS

7 tablespoons lightly salted butter, softened to room temperature

⅔ cup (packed) light brown sugar

1 large egg

½ teaspoon all-natural vanilla extract

⅔ cup gluten-free all-purpose flour blend (we've used Arrowhead Mills Gluten Free All Purpose Baking Mix)

1 teaspoon gluten-free baking powder

3 ounces good-quality white chocolate, chopped into small chunks, or white chocolate chips

¼ cup dried cherries

These make such lovely cookies to wrap up and give as little happies during the holidays. Kids love to help make these cookies, so if you have a special little helper, try enlisting him or her when baking. If you want to experiment with this cookie, try substituting your favorite nut and fruit combinations—macadamia nut and cranberry, perhaps. The cookies do expand quite a bit when cooking, so make sure these lil' babies have enough room to breathe on the baking sheets.

MAKES 18 TO 20 COOKIES, DEPENDING ON SIZE

STEPS

❶ Preheat the oven to 400°F. Line 2 large baking trays with parchment paper.

❷ In a large bowl, cream together the butter and sugar until light and fluffy, using either a hand-held or stand electric mixer.

❸ Add the egg and vanilla extract and beat well.

❹ In a separate small bowl, sift together the flour blend and baking powder.

❺ Add the dry ingredients to the butter mixture along with the chocolate chunks or chips and cherries. Mix all together well.

❻ Place heaping teaspoons of the cookie dough onto the prepared trays, making sure to leave enough room (at least 2 inches) for them to expand.

❼ Bake for 15 to 20 minutes, or until golden brown.

❽ Let cool directly on the parchment-lined trays and serve warm. They will crisp up when fully cooled. Store in an airtight container.

easy peasy chocolate fudge

INGREDIENTS

1 can (14 ounces) sweetened condensed milk

14 ounces plain milk chocolate, the higher the quality, the better

2 teaspoons all-natural vanilla extract

½ cup confectioner's sugar (powdered sugar), plus additional for garnish (optional)

Nuts or dried fruits of choice (optional)

This four-ingredient fudge is super easy to make, but it is so creamy and delicious that you'd think it took hours. It's terrific as a straightforward chocolate fudge or as a base for whatever other kinds of mix-ins you might prefer. Add walnuts or peanuts for a crunchy chocolate fudge or some dried cranberries or cherries for a fruity one. No matter how you make it, we are sure you will be happy with the result.

MAKES APPROXIMATELY 48 BITE-SIZE PIECES

STEPS

❶ Line an 8 × 8–inch glass baking dish with parchment paper and set aside.

❷ Using a double boiler or a heatproof bowl placed over a gently boiling pan of water, heat the condensed milk and chocolate, stirring, until the chocolate is completely melted and the mixture is thoroughly blended. Be sure to stir almost continuously to encourage even melting and to avoid burning the chocolate.

❸ Remove the melted liquid from the heat. Stir in the vanilla extract, confectioner's sugar, and any mix-ins you'd like.

❹ Spoon the mixture into the parchment-lined baking dish, making sure the surface is as level as possible. Place in the refrigerator and chill for at least 2 hours, or until firm.

❺ Once the fudge is sufficiently hardened, turn it out of the pan onto a cutting board. Gently peel the parchment away from the fudge and cut it into bite-size pieces. If desired, sprinkle with a bit of powdered sugar before serving.

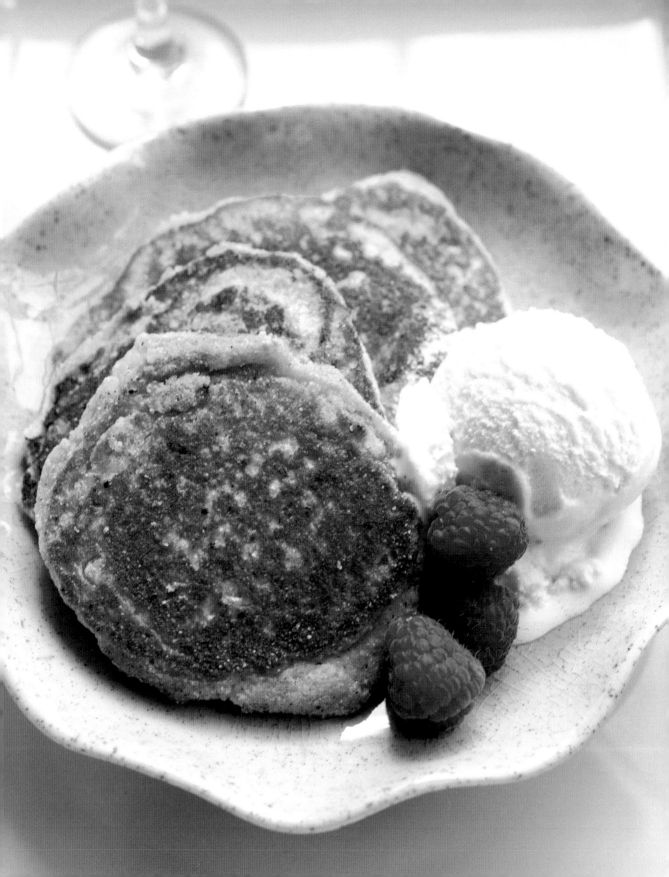

maple syrup johnnycakes
with ice cream

INGREDIENTS

1 cup gluten-free all-purpose flour blend (we've used Arrowhead Mills Gluten Free All Purpose Baking Mix)

2/3 cup cornmeal

3 tablespoons granulated sugar

1½ teaspoons gluten-free baking powder

½ teaspoon salt

2 large eggs, yolks and whites separated

¾ cup whole milk

¾ cup maple syrup

5 tablespoons (about 2/3 stick) unsalted butter, melted, plus additional for the griddle

Homemade Peach Ice Cream (recipe follows) or ice cream of your choice

Johnnycakes have been a long-standing tradition in New England, going all the way back to the Pilgrims. Traditionally made of cornmeal and water, the johnnycake can be dressed up in many ways. Our favorite version uses sugar and maple syrup to sweeten up the cake. It pairs very well with almost any flavor of ice cream, but we like them most when served warm with a fresh summer fruit ice cream like our Homemade Peach Ice Cream on page 216. Yum!

SERVES 6 TO 10, DEPENDING ON THE SIZE OF THE CORN CAKES

STEPS

1 Preheat the oven to 200°F.

2 In a large bowl, whisk together the dry ingredients.

3 In a separate bowl, whisk together the egg yolks, milk, and maple syrup to blend well. Add the mixture, along with the melted butter, to the dry ingredients and stir until well incorporated.

4 In a small bowl, using an electric mixer, beat the two egg whites until stiff peaks form. Gently fold the beaten whites into the batter.

5 Heat a griddle or skillet over medium heat and brush with butter. Pour ¼ to ½ cup batter onto the griddle for each cake. If you want to make smaller cakes and stack 4 or 5 of them per serving, use less batter per cake.

6 Cook for about 3 to 5 minutes, until bubbles form on the surface. Flip the johnnycakes and cook for another 2 to 3 minutes. As the cakes are done, remove from the griddle and place on a cookie sheet. Keep warm in a very low oven until ready to serve.

7 Depending on the size of the corn cakes, stack 2 to 5 on each plate and top with our Homemade Peach Ice Cream or flavor of your choice.

homemade peach ice cream

INGREDIENTS

1¼ to 1½ pounds ripe
    peaches

1 tablespoon lemon juice

1 cup heavy cream

½ cup whole milk

Seeds from ½ vanilla bean
    pod split lengthwise and
    scraped out

2 large egg yolks

⅓ cup granulated sugar

Pinch of salt

Nothing reminds us of summer more than fresh peach ice cream, especially when paired with our deliciously sweet Maple Syrup Johnnycakes (page 215)! It's important to use fresh peaches so you can use the skins and pits to infuse the cream-milk mixture. Although you can use frozen peaches, there will be no pits or skins for infusion: the ice cream will still be good but not as peachy. If you don't have an ice cream maker, you can simply mix everything together, pour it in a Pyrex dish, and freeze it. It won't turn out as creamy, but it will still taste fantastic!

MAKES 1 QUART

STEPS

❶ Fill a medium-size bowl with water and add ice cubes.

❷ Fill a medium-size saucepan with water and bring to a boil. Place the peaches in the boiling water for 1 minute. Transfer the peaches to the ice water to cool.

❸ Once the peaches are cool, drain again. Working with one peach at a time, remove the skin and pit, setting these aside in a small bowl.

❹ Cut each peach into medium-size chunks and toss in a separate bowl with the lemon juice. When all the peaches are in the bowl, refrigerate.

❺ In a medium-size saucepan over medium heat, bring the cream, milk, vanilla bean seeds, and peach skins and pits to a simmer. Remove immediately from the heat, cover, and let sit for approximately 20 minutes.

❻ While the cream mixture is infusing, thoroughly whisk together the egg yolks, sugar, and salt in a medium-size bowl.

❼ Strain the infused cream mixture into a second bowl.

❽ Stir half the infused cream into the egg yolk mixture to temper the yolks. Once the cream is incorporated, transfer the mixture along with the remaining infused cream to a clean saucepan.

9 Heat over medium heat, stirring constantly, until the mixture thickens slightly, about 5 minutes.

10 Strain the custard mixture into a clean bowl and refrigerate until thoroughly cooled, approximately 30 to 40 minutes.

11 Setting about a quarter of the peach chunks aside, puree the remainder in a blender along with half the cooled custard mixture. Pour the puree back into the bowl with the remaining custard and stir to blend.

12 Transfer the mixture to an ice cream maker and freeze according to the manufacturer's directions, folding in the peach chunks as instructed by the manufacturer as well. If you don't have an ice cream maker, simply fold the peach chunks into the mixture, pour it all into a large Pyrex dish, and freeze until firm, about 1 hour.

13 Transfer the ice cream to a plastic container, placing cling film directly on the ice cream's surface. Freeze until ready to use.

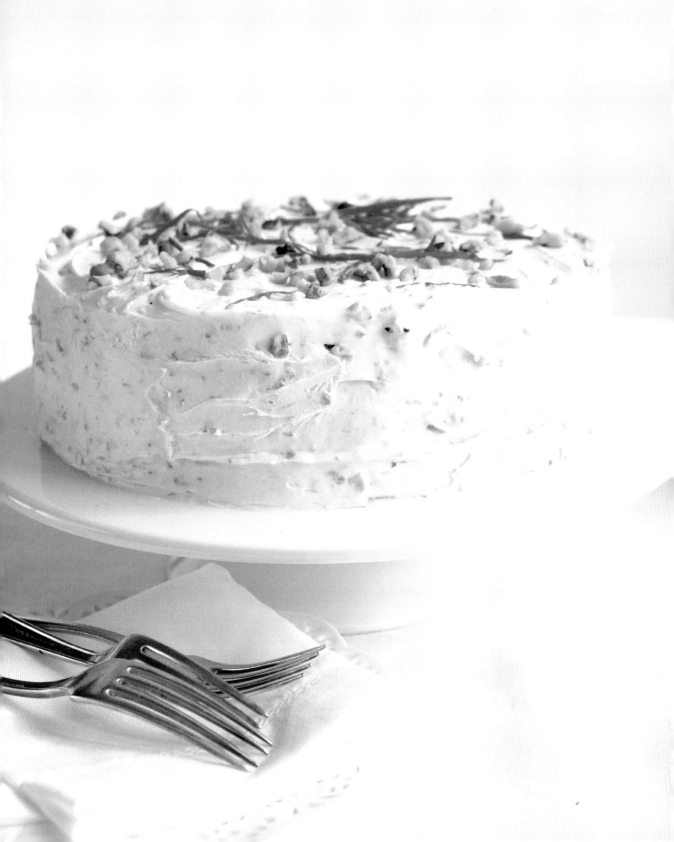

spiced carrot cake
with **sweet mascarpone frosting**

INGREDIENTS

12 tablespoons (1½ sticks) unsalted butter, softened to room temperature

1½ cups (packed) soft light brown sugar

6 large eggs

1 teaspoon all-natural vanilla extract

1½ cups gluten-free all-purpose flour blend (we've used Arrowhead Mills Gluten Free All Purpose Baking Mix)

1 heaping tablespoon plus 1 heaping teaspoon gluten-free baking powder

½ teaspoon ground cinnamon

1 teaspoon salt

½ cup almond meal/flour

2 cups finely grated carrot (about 2 large carrots, peeled)

1 cup walnuts or pecans (about 4 ounces), roughly chopped (optional)

2 tablespoons milk, any % fat you prefer

2 containers (14 ounces each) good-quality mascarpone cheese, softened to room temperature

½ cup confectioner's sugar (powdered sugar)

We've elevated the humble carrot cake to another level with our flavor-packed batter and sweet and creamy mascarpone frosting. This makes such a beautiful double-layered cake that it's almost too pretty to cut into . . . though you won't be able to resist doing so for very long. This is the perfect cake to make for a special occasion such as a birthday or tea party. It's both delicate and delicious. You can garnish the sides with a bit of grated carrot and chopped nuts, for an even more spectacular looking cake. You'll never see carrots the same way again.

SERVES 8 TO 10

STEPS

❶ Preheat the oven to 350°F. Grease and flour two 9-inch cake pans.

❷ In a large bowl, cream the butter and sugar until light and fluffy, using either a hand-held or stand electric mixer.

❸ Add the eggs and vanilla extract and beat until creamy.

❹ In a separate bowl, sift together the flour blend, baking powder, cinnamon, and salt.

❺ Stir in the almond meal/flour.

❻ Gently fold the dry ingredients into the butter mixture and blend until it becomes thick.

❼ Add 1¾ cups of the carrots, ⅔ cup of the walnuts (if using), and the milk and mix well.

❽ Spoon the batter into the prepared cake pans, dividing evenly.

❾ Bake for 35 to 40 minutes, or until a toothpick inserted in one of the layers comes away clean.

❿ Allow the layers to cool fully in the pans before trying to invert them.

(recipe continues)

⓫ While the layers are cooling, make the frosting. In a medium-size bowl, use a hand-held or stand electric mixer to mix the mascarpone cheese, confectioner's sugar, and ¼ cup of the remaining walnuts (if using) together until thoroughly incorporated. The consistency should be fluffy. Set aside.

⓬ Carefully invert one of the cake layers onto a serving plate or cake stand and frost the top with a small amount of the frosting; you need just a thin layer to act like a glue to hold the next layer on.

⓭ Carefully invert the second cake layer on top of the frosted layer. Generously cover the cake on the top and sides with the remaining frosting.

⓮ Sprinkle the remaining ¼ cup grated carrot and any remaining nuts over the top and sides the way you like.

⓯ Store the cake in the refrigerator until needed.

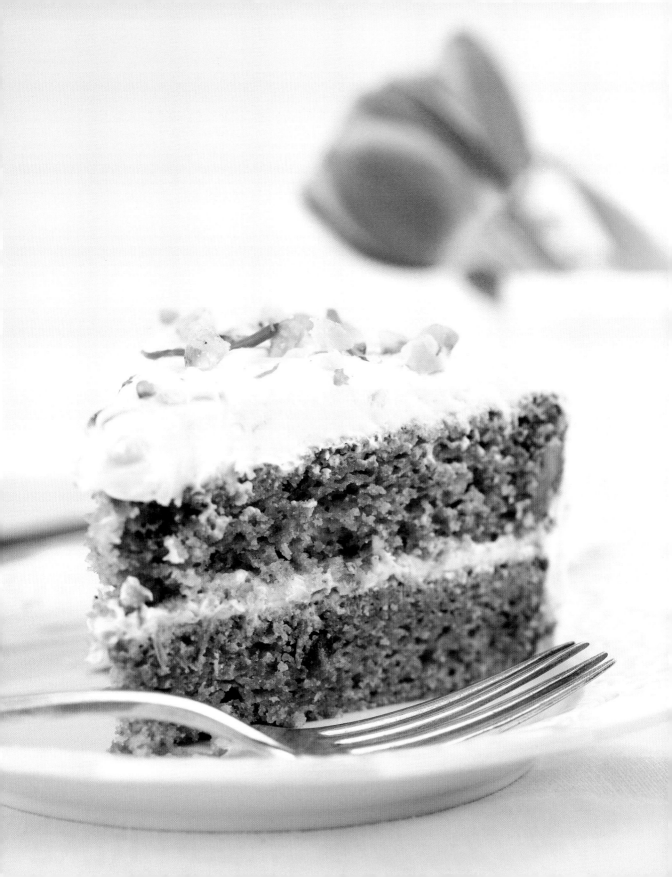

resources
and websites

This book just wouldn't be complete without a brief summary of helpful websites and resources. Again, these listings are not all-inclusive, but are some of the ones we find most helpful.

online resources for gluten-free products

www.celiac.com/glutenfreemall
(866)575-3720

They carry everything you can imagine—gluten-free frozen foods and pizza crusts, pantry staples, every type and shape of pasta, crackers, and condiments.

www.amazon.com

Amazon also has a huge selection of gluten-free products for sale, including lasagna sheets.

www.arrowheadmills.elsstore.com
(800)434-4246

Arrowhead Mills carries loads of fabulous gluten-free beans, rices, seeds, nut butters, flours, and baking mixes, including our personal favorite, which we use throughout the book, their Gluten Free All Purpose Baking Mix.

www.bobsredmill.com

This is a one-stop shop for all your gluten-free baking needs. They carry xanthan gum, almond meal/ flour, chickpea (gram) flour, tapioca flour, cornmeal, shredded coconut, and more.

www.wholefoodsmarket.com

You can log on and order from a store near you. This is a great place to buy crème fraîche, which we use throughout the book, along with countless other gluten-free essentials.

www.emerils.com

All of our dad's products, including his Original Essence Seasoning.

www.kalustyans.com
(212)685-3451

Kalustyan's is an amazing store based in NYC that carries every type of spice imaginable. They also carry Indian curry pastes, spices, chickpea (gram) flour, bean flours, rice flours, molasses, gluten-free tamari soy sauce, Thai fish sauce, coconut milk, and vermicelli rice noodles.

www.pataksusa.com
(800)726-3648

Patak's Original USA carries several gluten-free curry pastes and sauces.

www.englishteastore.com
(877)734-2458

Jilly's favorite place in the US to get all her British essentials, like ambrosia custard, Indian curry pastes, and Bisto Instant Gravy Granules, which happen to be gluten-free and with which, you'll have homemade gravy within 5 minutes.

www.clabbergirl.com
(812)232-9446

They carry both Clabber Girl and Rumford Gluten-Free Baking Powder and Corn Starch. Both are produced in a peanut-free facility, and you can buy in bulk.

www.againstthegraingourmet.com
(802)258-3838

This company makes the most delicious gluten-free baguettes, bagels, rolls, pizza shells, and more. Unfortunately, at this time they are unable to sell their products online directly to customers. However, you can ask your local grocery store manager to get in touch with them and find out how to carry their delicious products. It's easier than you think and so worth it!

helpful gluten free links/places doing great things

CELIAC DISEASE CENTER AT COLUMBIA UNIVERSITY
www.celiacdiseasecenter.columbia.edu

UNIVERSITY OF MARYLAND CELIAC CENTER FOR CELIAC RESEARCH
www.celiaccenter.org

UNIVERSITY OF CHICAGO CELIAC DISEASE CENTER
www.celiacdisease.net

AMERICAN CELIAC DISEASE CENTER
www.americanceliac.org

MAYO CLINIC
www.mayoclinic.com/health/celiac-disease

NATIONAL FOUNDATION FOR CELIAC AWARENESS
www.celiaccentral.org

CELIAC SPRUE ASSOCIATION
www.csaceliacs.org

CELIAC DISEASE FOUNDATION
www.celiac.org

fabulous gluten-free, allergy-related magazines we love

www.delightglutenfree.com
www.livingwithout.com
www.glutenfreeliving.com
www.allergicliving.com (click on the Celiac tab)

acknowledgments and thanks

jilly would like to thank:

First and foremost, I'd like to thank my parents, without whom I wouldn't be here today!

To my father, Emeril:
Daddio—thank you for instilling in me the true joy and passion of cooking and how special it is to share good food with the ones you love. I've learned so much from simply watching you. I hope we made you proud. All my love.

To my mother, Luz:
Momma—simply said, for everything I thank you. You have told me since I was a little girl to believe in my dreams, no matter how often those dreams have changed in my life.

I'd like to thank all my wonderful friends and family for their constant support and endless taste testing. In particular, the following:

To my incredible stepmother, Alden, for your undying support, advice, and love. You've taught me so very much. All my love and thanks always.

To my brother, E.J., and sister Meril. You are the light and laughter of my life and you inspire me daily.

To my sister Jessie for sharing this dream, for all your hard work and sacrifice to make this book happen. It's been a wild ride, but we did it!

To my wonderful brother-in-law, Steven. My frying partner in crime, I thank you for all your help and support during this process. We couldn't have done it without you.

To my gorgeous nephews Jude and J.P. I can't imagine you not being here and a part of it all.

To DS, thank you for your constant love and support. You make all the hard work worth it!

To my great-grandmother Cabral, thank you for all the beautiful memories and the joy you shared from feeding us all! These memories I will treasure forever.

To Grandma and Grandpa Kief and Grandma and Grandpa Lagasse. Thank you all for inspiring me to follow my heart and stomach!

To all my incredible aunts, uncles, and cousins, thank you for all the great times, wonderful memories, and the many traditions we have shared.

To everyone at 822: J, Drea, Nicole, Lizzie, and Melissa, you have inspired and supported me to follow this gluten-free dream for years! All my love and thanks to y'all.

To the Whittingtons: Jackie, Big Joe, Nathan, and Melly. This book wouldn't have happened without you. All my love and thanks.

To Tal Kohen, your support and humor have gotten me through.

To Ashley Denny, for letting me take over your kitchen and life for three months of testing and retesting recipes, I'm forever thankful.

To Shelly Montez, your incredible photography and styling made our dream that much closer to being actualized. Beyond grateful and thankful to you always.

To the Nemeth family: Tierney, Eric, and my darling Violet. Thank you for years of always being there and always being supportive no matter what my latest dream is!

To the Fontaines: Sareta, Danny, Diddy, and Zak. Finally, I did it! Thank you for years of laughter and friendship. Love you all so much.

To Nate and Kim, all my love and thanks.

jessie would like to thank:

My husband, Steven, for his unwavering support and unfaltering appetite through all these years.

My two wonderful sons, Jude and J.P., for reminding me every day how perfect life is!

My mom for giving my sons and me the greatest gift ever. Thanks for moving down the street!

My dad for his love, support, and valuable life lessons over all these years.

CiCi and Papa Derby, my other parents, for always being there for us.

Shelita Johnson, Gee Gee and Grandpa Kief, and Maw-Maw Patsy for their unending help with my kids, my house, and anything and everything else I can imagine. I could *never* have done this without you all and I am so very grateful!

My sister, Jill, for persevering and working so hard to get this done.

Marcus Azzarello for his tireless taste-testing and honest feedback.

Very special thanks go out from both of us to the following individuals who made this book possible:

To Nicole Hunn, who, thanks to a chance meeting, truly made this book happen and come to life.

To everyone at Foundry Media, especially Brandi Bowles. Brandi, thank you for taking our dream and turning it into our reality. You have quickly become a trusted sounding board and friend. For all your hard work, patience, and constant positivity, we will forever be thankful.

To everyone at Grand Central Publishing, especially Diana Baroni and Amanda Englander. Diana, thank you for seeing the bigger picture and taking a chance on us gals. We will always be grateful for this opportunity.

To our incredible photographer, Chris Granger. What an honor it was to have you on board this crazy gluten-free train. Your vision, talent, and humor were so appreciated every day. From day one, you just got it. Thank you.

To our talented food-styling team, Sara Essex Bradley and Rachel Witwer, thank you for all your hard work, vision, and not being afraid to get your hands dirty. Literally!

To everyone at Emeril's Homebase. In particular, special thanks go out to Tony Cruz, Charlotte Martory, Lolita Brooks, Paige Green, and chef David Slater, aka The Fig Man. Y'all rock!

A very special thank you to Maggie McCabe. All of this wouldn't have been possible without your calm and never-ending support. Love you, Maggarellos!

To Mark Stein, thank you for all your hard work and advice on this and every project.

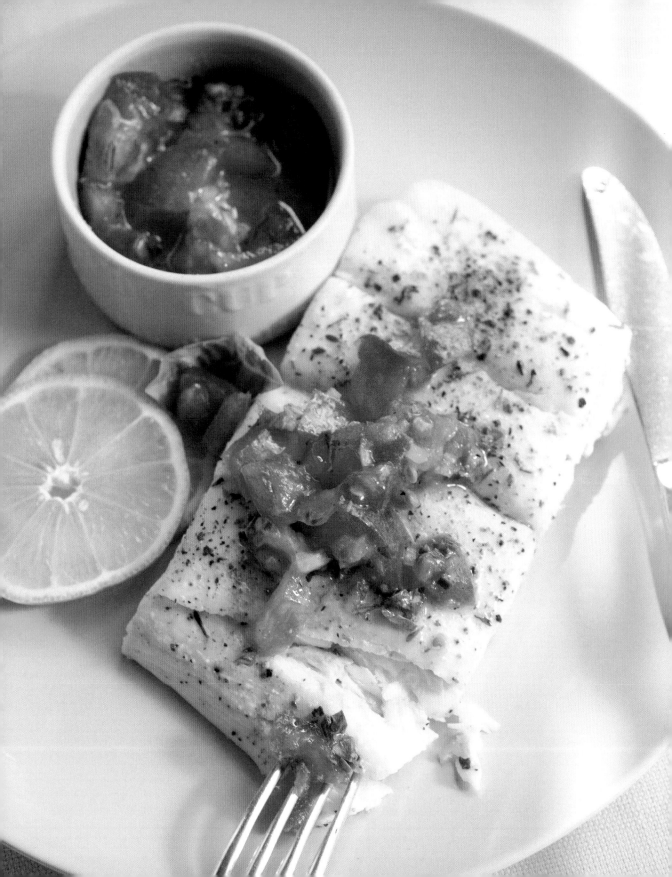

index

Page numbers of photographs appear in italics.